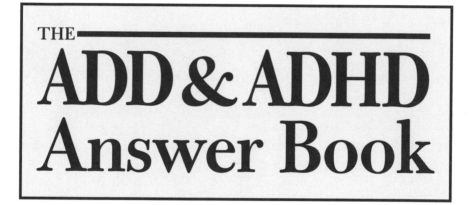

THE ADD & ADHD Answer Book

THE

ADD & ADHD
Answer Book

SUSAN ASHLEY, PhD

Published by Sourcebooks, Inc.
P.O. Box 4410, Naperville, Illinois   60567-4410
(630) 961-3900
Fax: (630) 961-2168
www.sourcebooks.com

Library of Congress Cataloging-in-Publication Data
Ashley, Susan, PhD.
  The ADD & ADHD answer book / Susan Ashley.
     p. cm.
  Includes bibliographical references and index.
  ISBN 1-4022-0549-X (alk. paper)
  1. Attention-deficit hyperactivity disorder--Popular works. I. Title.

RJ506.H9A327 2005
618.92'8589--dc22
                                        2005021669

Printed and bound in the United States of America.
BG 10 9 8

To parents searching for answers

Contents

Acknowledgments

There are many individuals who were helpful in the writing of this book whom I wish to thank.

I wish to thank the hundreds of children whom I have had the delight of knowing in my years of practice. They have been my greatest source of information. It is through them that I truly came to understand what it is like to be a child with AD/HD. I am honored by their parents for allowing me to enter their family and for trusting me with the most important person in their life.

My research assistant Tiffany Kleoni contributed to the development of this book in ways that cannot be measured. Her dedication, effort, and belief in this project helped immensely.

I am thankful for having the good fortune of working with Senior Editor Bethany Brown. She was instrumental in the birth and development of this book. Copy Editors Samantha Raue and Kelly Barrales-Saylor were most helpful in lending their eye for detail in the final stages of the book.

For their remarkable display of friendship to their schoolmates through the *Buddy Program*, I wish to thank Elliott and Aaron Stone, who are living role models for children to reach out to those in need.

Words cannot express my gratitude to my parents who provided me with the gift of a calm, structured, and predictable home life that has shaped not only what I teach parents in my practice, but also how I live my life.

My deepest appreciation to Stan for everything.

Introduction

The world of AD/HD is confusing and overwhelming. From the moment you suspect your child has AD/HD, you begin a journey that seems to have no road map. Once your child is diagnosed, the destination becomes even less clear.

- Does your child need to be tested?
- Should you try medication?
- What about special education?
- Is your daughter going to have low self-esteem?
- Will your son fail in school?

The list of questions goes on and on, but the answers are difficult to find.

Everywhere you turn for help, you are probably told that medication is the answer. Pediatricians tell you medication is the answer. Teachers tell you medication is the answer. Parents tell you medication is the answer. Surely you have wondered, "Isn't there something more than medication?"

You will not be told in this book that medication is the answer. While medication does have its usefulness, the primary goal of this book is to tell you the many, many ways you can help your child that have nothing to do with medication. Whether or not you give your child medication or are opposed to it does not change the fact that your child needs your help with homework, school, friendships, self-esteem, and behavior.

The ADD and ADHD Answer Book gives you the answers to your important questions. Over fifteen years in private practice specializing in evaluating and treating AD/HD has given me the inside perspective of what parents really want to know. The answers in this book are the same answers I would give to you if we were having a face-to-face consultation in my office. The answers are based on the current research and state-of-the-art psychological techniques.

This book differs from all other books about AD/HD because, like a dictionary, this book can be used as a reference. Over the years, as your child progresses through the various stages of this disorder, you will have *The ADD and ADHD Answer Book* on your reference shelf to find the answers to your new questions.

The ADD and ADHD Answer Book will transform you into a well-informed consumer. You will have extensive knowledge direct from a child psychologist who specializes in AD/HD. You will have straightforward, no holds barred, honest information about what you are likely to face over the years in raising your child with AD/HD. You will have the most current information based on research and clinical practice.

In writing *The ADD and ADHD Answer Book*, it is my hope that it becomes your guidebook and that you will use it frequently. I hope that you will turn to this book each time you have a question. It is my wish that you will use the numerous techniques in this book that I, and many child psychologists, have used over the years in treating children with AD/HD. I hope that you find the inspiration to apply the techniques, despite the tireless effort it requires on your part. While some of your reward for your hard work will come in the days, weeks, and months ahead, your true reward will come in the years ahead when you see your child succeed in school, find his place with friends, like who he has become, and find a passion in life that he can make his life's work.

Chapter 1

THE ABCs OF ADD AND ADHD

- What are the three types of ADD and ADHD?
- What are the symptoms of ADD?
- What does an ADD child look like in daily life?
- What other symptoms are associated with ADD?
- What are the symptoms of ADHD?
- What does an ADHD child look like in daily life?
- What other symptoms are associated with ADHD?
- How is the ADD child different from the ADHD child?
- Are ADD and ADHD real disorders?
- Is AD/HD over-diagnosed?
- Doesn't every child have symptoms of AD/HD?
- How can it be AD/HD when he can play video games for hours?
- Is there a difference between boys and girls who have AD/HD?
- Is AD/HD caused by something in the brain?
- Is AD/HD genetic?
- Can poor parenting cause AD/HD?
- What effect does the family environment have on AD/HD?
- Does watching television cause AD/HD?
- Do sugar and food allergies cause AD/HD?
- What other causes of AD/HD are suspected?
- Is there a cure for AD/HD?
- How is AD/HD treated?
- What can behavior modification do to help AD/HD?
- What can family therapy do to help?
- What can social skills group therapy do to help?
- What can individual therapy do to help?
- What treatments do not work?
- What should parents know when selecting treatment?

What are the three types of ADD and ADHD?

Before we can begin to answer the many questions about ADD and ADHD, it is important to learn the terminology and understand the difference between the language that parents use and the language you will hear from doctors.

The terminology of ADD and ADHD are defined in the *Diagnostic and Statistical Manual IV-TR* published by the American Psychiatric Association. ADD and ADHD have had various labels over the years, including minimal brain dysfunction and hyperkinesis. The current terminology for both ADD and ADHD is **Attention Deficit Hyperactivity Disorder**.

There are three types of Attention Deficit Hyperactivity Disorder:

Attention Deficit Hyperactivity Disorder, Primarily Inattentive Type. Children who have this type are inattentive and distractible. Even though the word "hyperactivity" is included in the label, there is no hyperactivity. This type is commonly called ADD.

Attention Deficit Hyperactivity Disorder, Primarily Hyperactive-Impulsive Type. Children with this disorder are overactive and impulsive. This type is most often called ADHD.

Attention Deficit Hyperactivity Disorder, Combined Type. These children are inattentive and distractible, as well as hyperactive and impulsive. This type is also referred to as ADHD.

What are the symptoms of ADD?

ADD is the inattentive type of ADHD. Children with ADD have six or more of the following symptoms, some of which start before they reach seven years of age:

- Forgetful in daily activities
- Poor attention to details and careless mistakes in schoolwork and homework
- Easily distracted by extraneous stimuli
- Trouble sustaining attention
- Loses things necessary for tasks or activities
- Dislikes and is reluctant to exert sustained mental effort
- Does not follow through on instructions and fails to finish chores and schoolwork
- Difficulty organizing tasks and activities
- Does not seem to listen when spoken to directly

Because toddlers and early elementary school children are not expected to sustain attention for long periods, or to keep track of their own belongings, ADD often does not become problematic until third or fourth grade when children are expected to function more independently.

Symptoms must be present for at least six months and appear in more than one setting. Children's symptoms are most commonly seen at home and at school, but they are also likely to show up in other settings where attention is needed such as church or temple, music lessons, and sport activities.

What does an ADD child look like in daily life?

The ADD child is usually a cooperative child who simply is unable to function well in situations that require sustained attention and organization. They typically are nice children who are not outright defiant, but just have great trouble finding the mental energy it takes to pay attention to things that are not especially exciting to them.

These children are forgetful in everyday routines, seeming to have never heard the rules and routine before. They will carelessly add when they should subtract and multiply when they should divide. They are more interested in the noise outside than listening to the teacher. While it is no trouble to play video games for hours, doing five math problems causes tears and tantrums. They lose their backpack, homework, jacket, and lunchbox. Chores and homework rarely get finished without great effort by parents. Their desk, backpack, and bedroom look like mystery science projects you are scared to go near. All this goes on while they seem to be happily daydreaming the day away. As long as no one is asking them to do something, they are fine. It is when it is time to pay attention and complete tasks that the trouble surfaces.

What other symptoms are associated with ADD?

If the only problems caused by ADD were that the child was forgetful, distractible, and inattentive, it would not be such a difficult disorder. The real difficulty in raising a child with ADD is that the symptoms cause a host of other very difficult problems. Not liking to exert mental effort does not cause any problems until it is time to do homework. Knowing that he will miss out on fun each afternoon because he has homework leads the ADD child to lie about having homework, hide the homework, and purposely forget his schoolbooks. Needing to focus on homework and think about a subject that the child finds boring leads the ADD child to procrastinate, argue, cry, throw tantrums, and in more severe cases, hit parents and break things in the house. Homework that should take fifteen minutes can take two hours, interfering with playtime, dinner, and bath and bedtime. Simply being inattentive can be very damaging to family life with daily upsets and arguments that can last several hours. The daily struggles between parent and child erode the relationship, prevent fun time with one another, and cause mutual resentment. Life during the school year can be very unhappy for both the parents and the child.

What are the symptoms of ADHD?

ADHD is the hyperactive and impulsive type of ADHD. Children with ADHD have six or more of the following symptoms, some of which start before they reach seven years of age:

- Talks excessively
- Fidgets or squirms in seat
- On the go or acts as if driven by a motor
- Leaves seat when expected to remain seated
- Runs or climbs when it is inappropriate
- Difficulty playing quietly
- Interrupts or intrudes on others
- Blurts out answers before questions are complete
- Difficulty waiting for turn

ADHD often appears before the child starts school. As early as toddler years, these children will be easily visible to others as behaving differently from other children their age. Once the ADHD child starts preschool or kindergarten, their teacher is likely to report to parents their observation of many of the symptoms. Expulsion from preschool is often the first indicator of ADHD.

Symptoms must be present for a minimum of six months and must be seen in more than one setting. The symptoms are most commonly seen at home and school, but will surely be displayed in restaurants, grocery stores, movie theatres, and any place where it is not acceptable to be loud and active.

What does an ADHD child look like in daily life?

The ADHD child is a high maintenance child who requires almost constant supervision. They are difficult children who do not like to sit down, wait their turn, or be quiet. As toddlers, they run away from parents in stores, jump up and down in restaurant booths, and scream in church. In preschool, they run around almost constantly, grab toys, do not listen to teachers, and seem to never tire out. In elementary school, they wander around the classroom, disturb the other students, shout out answers, and talk too much. On the playground, they grab the ball, disrupt games, and shove their way in line. At home, constant battles ensue over every minor request and rule. Wherever they are, they talk too much, too loudly, too often, and in places where they should be quiet. They have trouble settling down and playing quietly; however, if they enjoy television, computers, or video games, they are able to sit peacefully for long stretches at a time.

The ADHD child tries the patience of everyone. They frequently are rejected by their peers, especially as they get older. They frustrate their parents, teachers, coaches, and babysitters.

What other symptoms are associated with ADHD?

The symptoms of ADHD alone are enough to make life very difficult for both the child and parents. Because the ADHD child is so hard to manage, simply getting through each day can be a challenge. Arguments occur with simple requests, causing parents to resort to yelling in order to get their child to listen. From the child refusing to get out of bed in the morning to refusing to get back in at night, the day is filled with continual power struggles. Crying, screaming, and throwing tantrums are frequent events. Reports sent home from school are common occurrences. Impulsive actions on the playground can cause the ADHD child to get into physical fights with peers, be rejected, and have no friends. The ADHD child is often hard to satisfy and for some children, no matter how much they are given, it is never enough. They negotiate, argue, and throw tantrums to get what, they want and have stamina that wears most parents out. In order to gain peace in the home, parents may be tempted to give in to many of the ADHD child's demands, allowing the child to escape bedtime, chores, and having to comply with rules. The daily negativity in the life of the ADHD child can lead to sadness and low self-esteem.

How is the ADD child different from the ADHD child?

ADHD children are very different from ADD children in the early years. Even though it is rare for a toddler to be diagnosed with ADHD, in hindsight, some parents of ADHD children report that their child was difficult from the time they could walk. In contrast, ADD children usually do not display symptoms in the years before they go to school.

Once in kindergarten, the ADHD child may have trouble sitting still, following directions, and controlling his over-activity. The ADD child behaves well in kindergarten, but may display mild troubles with paying attention.

As the ADHD child moves into first and second grade, behavior management becomes more difficult at home and school. Social problems are more apparent. The ADD child continues to behave well, but slowly shows developing struggles with homework and paying attention in class.

By third or fourth grade, both disorders are usually apparent to parents and teachers. The ADHD child often is having many behavior problems by this time. His home life and school life are both difficult to manage. The ADD child visibly struggles with class work and homework and many of his attention difficulties are now displayed in problematic behavior.

Are ADD and ADHD real disorders?

This is a question of popular debate. Skeptics state that the disorder is made up by a high-pressured American society that expects more from children at a younger age. Many parents, fathers in particular, are prone to say that society simply forgot what it was like to be an active child—a sort of "boys will be boys" viewpoint. Others campaign that overcrowded schools have made teachers intolerant of children who are a bit "different," and those who do not fit in are now labeled as disordered. These arguments are fiercely challenged by parents raising a child with AD/HD. Teachers, pediatricians, and psychologists working with these children will also substantiate the existence of the disorders.

Hundreds of published studies provide strong evidence for the existence of ADD and ADHD. The current scientific belief is that AD/HD is a "biopsychosocial" disorder that likely has its roots in the interaction of human biology, psychology, and the social environment. While the cause has yet to be found, the reality of AD/HD has long been answered. AD/HD is an extreme manifestation of normal behaviors, just as normal sadness, when extreme, is called depression. AD/HD, like many mental disorders, is a group of symptoms that, when manifested together frequently, intensely, and severely, presents as a disorder.

Is AD/HD over-diagnosed?

Public perception is that the number of children diagnosed with AD/HD is growing each year. In the previous decade, it was estimated that between 3 to 5 percent of children were affected by AD/HD. Current estimates range from 6 to 9 percent. Is the disorder actually becoming more frequent or are professionals becoming more skilled at diagnosis?

Researchers argue that the disorder itself is not increasing, rather, as science learns more about AD/HD, doctors are becoming more skilled in detecting it. Parents and teachers are becoming more knowledgeable with the attention given to AD/HD in newspapers, magazines, and television, and are, therefore, more likely to refer a child for an evaluation.

Another common public perception is that AD/HD is primarily an American disorder.

However, research demonstrates that AD/HD is a disorder that exists across the world. Numerous countries, including Great Britain, Japan, China, Hong Kong, and Germany, among others, have similar or even greater rates of AD/HD than the USA.

Despite the research refuting over-diagnosis, it is important for parents to be aware that some teachers are more likely to suspect AD/HD and some professionals are more prone to render the diagnosis. Parents should therefore feel comfortable seeking a second opinion.

Doesn't every child have symptoms of AD/HD?

When you read down the list of symptoms of AD/HD, it sure seems like it describes almost every child. All children, and even adults for that matter, exhibit some symptoms of AD/HD at some time.

If everyone displays some of the symptoms some of the time, how do you tell who truly has the disorder? The key to distinguishing typical behaviors from the diagnosable condition is that the symptoms must be *excessive*. According to the *Diagnostic and Statistical Manual IV-TR (DSM-IV-TR)* the manual mental health professionals use to make diagnoses, the symptoms must be "inconsistent with developmental level." It is not enough to go down the list and check off all the behaviors you have seen your child exhibit. You must check off only those symptoms that are excessive when compared to others your child's age and developmental level.

It is also not enough that the child merely displays the symptoms. The *DSM-IV- TR* also states that the symptoms must be "maladaptive." This means the symptoms must cause significant problems. It is not enough to simply have the symptoms. They must cause "significant impairment" in the child's functioning. Thus, the "A" student who daydreams in class is not going to be diagnosed with ADD because his inattentiveness is not negatively impairing his academic functioning.

How can it be AD/HD if he can play video games for hours?

The AD/HD child's ability to play computer and video games or watch television for hours baffles parents, leading them to mistakenly see this as proof that their child can concentrate and therefore does not have AD/HD. The important distinction is not that the child cannot pay attention, but that the child has great difficulty sustaining attention in tasks that require mental effort. In essence, when the child enjoys the task, he finds it easy. If the child does not like the task and finds it difficult and/or boring, he must exert mental effort to focus and complete the task. The child does not choose whether or not to exert mental effort; he has far greater difficulty staying focused and ignoring distractions on more difficult and less exciting tasks. The same is true for most people in general. It is easier to attend to pleasurable and interesting things than it is to boring things. The difference is that the average person is able to exert the mental effort despite how boring the material is, whereas the AD/HD child is not.

Is there a difference between boys and girls who have AD/HD?

Boys have ADHD approximately 4 to 9 times more often than girls do. ADD, on the other hand, tends to be present more equally between boys and girls.

Both boys and girls with AD/HD are generally less well liked by their peers and more prone to report having fewer friends than their non-AD/HD counterparts. Girls with AD/HD are more accurate and honest in their self-perceptions than are AD/HD boys. Girls report more problems with self-esteem, depression, family relationships, and peer rejection than boys. In stark contrast to the honest disclosure by girls, however, boys tend to overestimate their performance. They rate themselves as better at schoolwork, behavior, and peer relationships than their teachers rate them. Boys either are in denial or use an inflated sense of self to protect themselves against the depression that would surface if they were to acknowledge their deficits. Girls' self-awareness may be the reason they have three times more depression than AD/HD boys.

Is AD/HD caused by something in the brain?

Brain structure and functioning are suspected as playing a role in causing both ADD and ADHD. Through modern technology and techniques of magnetic resonance imaging (MRI), positron emission tomography (PET), and single photon emission computed tomography (SPECT), researchers can examine the brain.

Researchers have found the brain volume of AD/HD children to be 3 to 4 percent smaller in the frontal lobes. The frontal lobes of the brain, located near our foreheads, are responsible for problem solving, planning, understanding cause and effect, and controlling impulses—all problem areas for AD/HD children.

Glucose, the main source of brain energy, is also thought to be different in people with AD/HD. Adult studies have found that the brain areas that control attention use less glucose than those without the disorder, suggesting that the AD/HD brain is less active in some areas.

The **dopamine hypothesis** is one of the leading theories about AD/HD. Dopamine is thought to be important in increasing motivation and alertness, key weaknesses for AD/HD children. Dopamine is also thought to reduce appetite and cause insomnia, common side effects of stimulant medication. Since AD/HD responds well to stimulant medications by increasing the availability of the neurotransmitter dopamine, researchers are examining whether a deficit of dopamine is the cause.

Is AD/HD genetic?

It is common to hear that AD/HD is inherited or genetic. While scientists are very active in studying this theory, at this point no gene has been found. However, there is good reason for the research to continue, as these disorders do run in families. Approximately one half of parents with AD/HD have a child with the disorder. Anywhere from 10 to 35 percent of close relatives of children with AD/HD also have the disorder.

First-degree relatives of children with AD/HD and antisocial behavior are more likely to have AD/HD when compared to relatives of children with AD/HD without antisocial behavior.

Twin studies have found a greater likelihood of both twins having this disorder if they are identical twins that share 100 percent of their genes, than if they are fraternal twins who share 50 percent of their genes on average. If one identical twin has AD/HD, chances are 50 to 80 percent that the other identical twin will also have the disorder. Adoption studies have shown that the biological parents of children with AD/HD are more likely to have AD/HD than the adoptive parents, again suggesting genetic influences. Overall, there is strong evidence that AD/HD may be inherited.

Can poor parenting cause AD/HD?

One of the first questions parents ask after finding out their child has AD/HD is, "Did I do something to cause this?" The answer is "No." Poor parenting cannot cause AD/HD. Nothing a parent does or fails to do can cause AD/HD. You can breathe a sigh of relief knowing that the research undeniably shows that parents do not cause AD/HD.

While poor parenting does not *cause* these disorders, it is important that parents know that poor parenting can make the situation worse. Parents of AD/HD children have been found to be more rejecting, coercive, negative, and critical. Mothers of sons with AD/HD tend to be less approving, and more demanding. When AD/HD coexists with Oppositional Defiant Disorder (ODD), parenting becomes even more problematic, with parents being far more inconsistent and failing to work together.

These findings do not mean that the poor parenting causes AD/HD; in fact, it is most likely that having a child with AD/HD causes these types of reactions in parents and not the other way around. Effective parenting can decrease the negative cycle between the child's symptoms and parents' negative reaction.

To learn more about parenting, read Chapter 6: Parenting Rules, Routine, and Rewards.

What effect does the family environment have on AD/HD?

Just as poor parenting does not cause AD/HD, neither does the family environment.

The family environment, however, does have an effect on the AD/HD child. Research has consistently found a link between marital conflict and behavior problems in children. When children have AD/HD coexisting with another disorder, such as ODD, the parents experience more conflict over childrearing than parents of children with just AD/HD. Parents' inability or lack of effort to structure or regulate their child's behavior has been found to be significantly higher in families with an AD/HD child.

The family environment of AD/HD children has been found to show a reciprocal effect whereby the behavior of the children affects parenting style and parenting style in turn affects children's behavior. AD/HD children are less responsive to parental commands. Parents in turn are more controlling, critical, and punitive than parents of non-AD/HD children. Mothers give fewer positive responses to their AD/HD children and spend more time trying to direct, control, and structure their children's activities.

Family environments of AD/HD children tend to be less supportive, less cohesive, and less expressive. Parenting skills of those raising AD/HD children are generally weaker and parents have trouble managing rules, using reinforcers, and monitoring their child's behavior.

Does watching television cause AD/HD?

The theory behind television causing decreased attention span is the high level of rapid stimulation television provides in comparison to everyday life and the ordinary pace of the classroom. Due to research demonstrating that intense auditory and visual stimulation has a significant influence on brain development, the American Pediatric Association recommends that parents exercise caution in allowing children less than two years old to watch television.

Research has found a connection between early television exposure at age one to three years and later attention problems at seven years. The attention problems found in 10 percent of the 2,600 children studied were not indicative of AD/HD, but suggestive of problems with difficulty concentrating, becoming easily confused, impulsive, restless, and troubled by obsessions. Children who watched the most television had a 28 percent higher chance of having later problems with attention.

Before you rush to turn off the television, be aware that these findings do not mean that television causes attention problems or AD/HD. It is possible that early television watching leads to attention problems, or it could be that children with early problems with attention are more likely to be allowed by their parents to watch television as a means to keep them stimulated and quiet.

Do sugar and food allergies cause AD/HD?

While one theory is that AD/HD is caused by deficiencies in diet, another school of thought is that it is caused by dietary excess. Pediatric allergist Benjamin Feingold, MD, initiated the concern about artificial additives in our food in the 1970s. His elimination diet omitted dyes, artificial flavorings, and salicylates, and claimed to result in dramatic improvement in behavior. Numerous follow-up studies failed to find Feingold's theory to hold true for a large number of children.

Food allergies have long been suspected as a contributor to behavior problems as well. Common culprits of milk, nuts, and wheat have been linked to behavioral disturbance in some children. Eliminating the offending foods has been shown to improve mood, sleep, and some behaviors in a small percentage of allergic children. Elimination diets, however, are not regarded by physicians as an effective treatment for AD/HD.

Sugar is perhaps the most commonly accused food of causing hyperactivity. Repeated research has failed to find this to be true, but the myth persists to this day.

What other causes of AD/HD are suspected?

In the absence of finding an exact cause, researchers continue to expand their area of focus beyond genetics and brain structure. Vaccines have been suspected of being linked to a variety of neurodevelopmental disorders, including AD/HD. One large-scale study with more than 152,000 children, however, did not find evidence that there is any correlation between the agents in vaccines and AD/HD.

The mental health of mothers is another suspected cause of AD/HD. In a study of 9,500 families, mothers raising children with AD/HD were four times more likely to have a chronic and serious mental health condition. This does not mean that mothers' mental health causes AD/HD, but that the two are somehow connected. It could be that having an AD/HD child causes mothers to develop mental health disorders.

Maternal smoking during pregnancy has been shown in some studies to have a relationship to the later development of AD/HD. In some studies, injuries during birth have been found to be more common in children with AD/HD than those without the disorder. Extremely low birth weight has been found to be associated with AD/HD in some studies, but not in others. Exposure to environmental contaminants is being studied as a possible cause.

These particular theories have resulted in conflicting results and further studies are needed.

Is there a cure for AD/HD?

Unfortunately, there is no known cure for ADD or ADHD and nothing in the current research suggests that a cure will be found in the near future. ADD and ADHD are considered chronic disorders that last at least until adolescence. Even with the best treatment, medication, parenting, schooling, and therapy, ADD and ADHD are not curable.

It used to be thought that AD/HD was cured by children simply "growing out of it" by the time they finished high school. That notion has been abandoned, as research is finding that more children than previously thought retain the disorder during their adult years. Current research estimates that only about one third of children with the disorder overcome it. Two thirds are now thought to retain the disorder throughout their adult years.

Given the lack of a cure, treatment for AD/HD focuses on managing the symptoms rather than curing them. Once parents accept the long-term nature of the disorder and quit looking for a magic cure, it is easier to settle into management.

How is AD/HD treated?

AD/HD can be treated with a variety of interventions. A multi-modal treatment plan has been shown to be the most effective, rather than simply choosing one form of intervention.

Behavior modification is used to help manage the majority of the symptoms of AD/HD. Behavior modification is most successful when the child has a program for home and for school. Social skills training is used to help the AD/HD child gain self-awareness and learn new skills to increase his or her ability to make and keep friends. Special education and/or tutoring are used to increase the child's learning and success in school. Medication is used to decrease inattention, hyperactivity, and impulsivity.

Because the symptoms of AD/HD affect the child in every avenue of his or her life, treatment must address each of these avenues. Interventions need to be designed for home, school, playground, after school, homework, dinnertime, chores, bath time, and bedtime.

AD/HD is a full-time disorder that runs twenty-four hours a day, seven days a week, 365 days a year. Treatment needs to keep up with the disorder. Treatment options include:

- Behavior modification
- Family therapy
- Social skills group therapy
- Individual therapy
- Medication
- Special education
- Tutoring
- Organizational skills

What can behavior modification do to help AD/HD?

Behavior modification is the systematic use of rules, rewards, consequences, and privileges based upon the child's compliance. Research shows behavior modification to be the most effective tool in managing the AD/HD child's problematic behavior.

Behavior modification works on the principle that behaviors will increase if they are reinforced and decreased if they are punished. Using praise, stickers, points, prizes, and privileges for appropriate behavior results in significant increases in desirable behaviors. When these rewards and privileges are withheld, noticeable decreases in undesirable behaviors occur.

The use of behavior modification creates a highly structured environment for the child where the expectations for behavior are very clear. Exact rewards and punishments are spelled out ahead of time so that the child is fully aware of what will happen if they engage in certain behaviors. This allows for a predictable daily life for both parents and child.

Behavior modification is the best tool parents can learn in order to manage their child's symptoms. By far, however, it is also the most work for the parent, as it requires consistency and predictability every single day of the week, month, and year.

To learn how to use behavior modification, read Chapter 6: Parenting Rules, Routine, and Rewards.

What can family therapy do to help?

AD/HD children are high maintenance. They exhaust their parents and irritate their siblings. Parents find themselves in frequent conflict with one another as they argue over whether or not the AD/HD child misbehaved on purpose and whether or not he should be punished. Just getting the AD/HD child through the day places an enormous strain on the family. Parents are often so exhausted mentally, emotionally, and physically that they have little energy left for their partner and other children. Spouses feel neglected and siblings feel jealous of the attention the AD/HD child receives. Family therapy addresses these frustrations and helps the family live a calmer life that is not dominated by the AD/HD child.

Marital relationships can become strained from the strife the AD/HD child causes. It is typical for parents to argue over parenting techniques. It also is not strange for parents to lose their identity as a couple in their attempt to help their child. Couples therapy can help parents become a unified team and learn how to use the same parenting goals and skills. It also helps to renew their relationship as an adult couple, separate from their role as parents.

What can social skills group therapy do to help?

Everywhere the AD/HD child goes, he is identified as "the problem child." Social skills group therapy eliminates that feeling by providing a sense of belonging and acceptance by his peers. Often times, social skills group therapy is the first time the AD/HD child realizes he is not the only one struggling with behavior, school, and friendships. Being with similar peers helps the child feel as if he is not so different after all.

Social skills group therapy for AD/HD children teaches social skills reinforced by role-playing and repeated practice of the learned skills. Increasing self-esteem is a primary goal of group therapy.

Children are praised and reinforced for appropriate social behavior and given plenty of opportunity to receive positive feedback from the group leader and group members.

Group therapy provides a safe place for AD/HD children to express feelings and talk about the hurt they feel from being rejected and teased by their peers. Through learning, role-playing, feedback, and practice, they gain awareness of the behaviors that lead to social rejection and learn positive ways to interact with their peers so they can eventually gain acceptance and develop lasting friendships. To learn more about social skills read Chapter 8: Social Skills.

What can individual therapy do to help?

Individual therapy for AD/HD is probably the least effective treatment. The AD/HD child has little self-awareness and is not capable of observing himself, evaluating his behavior, and reflecting on whether or not his interactions with others were appropriate. The AD/HD child does not come to therapy saying that he realizes he has poor social skills, is not compliant with his parents, exasperates others, and therefore he wants help. Instead, he is prone to blame others, take no responsibility, have no clue as to why he is socially on the outskirts, why his siblings are mad at him, and why his parents are always yelling at him. Without the ability to identify and acknowledge their behavior and social problems, AD/HD children cannot make much use of what individual therapy has to offer. Group therapy is therefore a far more effective format for helping AD/HD children, as it provides the therapist with direct observation of the child's behavior in a group setting and demonstrates exactly how the child behaves.

Individual therapy can be helpful in addressing the negative mood and self-esteem that typically coexists with AD/HD. It is also the treatment of choice for secondary disorders such as depression, anxiety, trauma, or effects of divorce.

What treatments do not work?

In an effort to find a cure, and, unfortunately, probably find money too, several methods of treating AD/HD are currently being used which have no scientific support. Living with an AD/HD child is incredibly difficult, making it easy to see how parents fall prey to "revolutionary" methods that promise to change their child's behavior forever. Parents must know that if there were a cure, professionals specializing in AD/HD would be using it. Do not rely on advertising materials as evidence of success, as there is no one scrutinizing their claims. If a method has not been proven repeatedly in scientific journals to effectively reduce some of the symptoms of AD/HD, parents should stay away. Some of these methods can waste valuable time, money, and emotions, and others can actually be potentially dangerous. Any serious consideration of these methods must be discussed with your child's medical doctor. Some of the latest unproven methods advertised include:

- Megavitamin therapy—mega doses of vitamins and/or minerals
- Eye movement desensitization—eye exercises
- Herbal remedies—ingesting herbs
- Sound treatment—listening to voice, music, and chants
- Hypnotherapy—hypnosis
- Biofeedback/Neurofeedback—changing brain waves with computer feedback
- Sensory integration therapy—exposure to extrasensory stimulation
- Homeopathy—plant, mineral, and animal extracts
- Neural organization—adjustment of the cranial bones

What should parents know when selecting treatment?

Treatment options can be confusing and difficult to weed out the authentic from the snake oil. Parents must become informed consumers and know what the research says about treatment for AD/HD. Research has supported for decades that the use of medication and behavior modification are effective in reducing symptoms. Various methods of psychotherapy are effective in helping with the related problems that surface because of the disorder. Use common sense and if it sounds too good to be true, it is.

Perhaps the most difficult aspect of AD/HD is the lack of a cure. Treatment is long term and works best when parents stick with an experienced team of professionals who can help over the years as the child changes throughout his development.

When making decisions about treatment, keep in mind:

- There is no cure for AD/HD
- We do not know what causes AD/HD
- Treatment is to reduce and manage symptoms, not cure the disorder
- AD/HD lasts at least until adolescence
- Treatment is long term, usually years
- Many children have symptoms throughout adulthood
- Medication must not be the only form of treatment
- Behavioral treatment is a first line of treatment, with or without medication
- Parents must be active participants in their child's treatment

Chapter 2

GETTING YOUR CHILD EVALUATED

- What symptoms signal that my child should be evaluated?
- When is it time to get my child evaluated?
- Is a diagnosis necessary?
- How do I find a doctor?
- What type of doctor should evaluate my child?
- What should parents know about pediatricians?
- What should parents know about developmental pediatricians?
- What should parents know about child psychiatrists?
- What should parents know about pediatric neurologists?
- What should parents know about clinical psychologists?
- What should parents know about pediatric neuropsychologists?
- What should parents know about educational psychologists?
- What should parents look for in choosing a doctor?
- What medical tests are used to diagnose AD/HD?
- What psychological or educational tests are used to diagnose AD/HD?
- Do children behave differently in a one-on-one testing situation?
- If I have my child tested, what tests should be used?
- What use do I make out of the test results?
- What information can an IQ test provide?
- What information can academic achievement tests provide?
- What information can personality testing provide?
- How often should testing be done?
- What information can school achievement tests provide?
- What information can report cards provide?
- Can a diagnosis be made from a behavior checklist?
- Can a diagnosis of AD/HD be made from a computerized test?
- What information should I tell the doctor?
- What records should I give to the doctor?
- What questions will the doctor ask me about my child?
- What if the evaluation is inconclusive?

What symptoms signal that my child should be evaluated?

The majority of parents, upon learning that their child has AD/HD, reports suspecting it for several years. Parents of ADHD children often recall that their child was displaying symptoms as young as two years old. Early warning signs include intense tantrums, being in constant motion, and great difficulty taking the child in public. For preschool children, expulsion is a sure indicator that the child needs to be evaluated. Preschool children who repeatedly hit others, grab toys, refuse to sit in circle time, or take a nap, warrant an evaluation. Some children with ADHD may not have troubles surface until kindergarten, especially if they did not attend preschool. Reports from the teacher that the child literally roams around the classroom, will not sit down for long, disrupts story time, hits peers, and will not follow rules, should prompt an evaluation.

ADD symptoms surface later than ADHD. More severe forms of ADD begin to surface in first and second grade when the child is unable to listen, remain seated, and produce small amounts of work. Milder forms of ADD may not surface until third or fourth grade, when the child is unable to complete worksheets in the classroom and homework takes several hours to complete.

When is it time to get my child evaluated?

The time to seek an evaluation is as soon as you begin to suspect that your child does not function or behave like other children his age. Observations from teachers, relatives, friends, and other parents may be your first indication that your child may have AD/HD. Repeated feedback from others, even if you don't agree, should warrant an evaluation. Even if a diagnosis is not determined at the time, symptoms can be defined and interventions can begin. Research repeatedly and consistently shows that the earlier the detection and treatment, the better the long term outcome for the child and family.

Unfortunately, the majority of parents are reluctant to seek an evaluation and hold out hope that the child will grow out of the symptoms, believing it to be a phase. The most common age for parents to seek an evaluation is at nine years old, the fourth grade. When interviewed, virtually every parent can report symptoms that began years ago; however, they were hoping they would disappear. Only when faced with severe symptoms or expulsions do many parents relent and seek help. This is unfortunate because many years are wasted that the child could have been receiving interventions.

Is a diagnosis necessary?

A diagnosis describes a group of symptoms and provides a concise vocabulary for educators, parents, physicians, and mental health professionals to use. Of course, a diagnosis does not tell all there is to know about a child. Yet, knowing a child has been diagnosed with AD/HD provides a tremendous amount of information. It helps explain behavior, increasing understanding of why the child is behaving in certain patterns. A formal diagnosis is not always necessary. If symptoms can be identified and interventions planned, a diagnosis does not have to be made. However, there are situations when a diagnosis is required. When seeking reimbursement from insurance, a diagnosis is always required. Special education services require the presence of a disorder that impairs learning. Obtaining medication requires a diagnosis.

Some children have symptoms of AD/HD that are not severe enough to meet criteria for the diagnosis of AD/HD. These children can nonetheless benefit from an evaluation and interventions designed to address their symptoms.

How do I find a doctor?

Finding an experienced physician or mental health professional with expertise in evaluating AD/HD is one of the most important decisions you will make as a parent. Some parents shy away from professionals who specialize in AD/HD, believing the expert will see the disorder in every child. This fear results in evaluations performed by less experienced professionals who are unfamiliar with AD/HD. An expert in AD/HD will not diagnose AD/HD simply because that is their expertise. They have seen hundreds of children with AD/HD and have seen the infinite number of ways the symptoms manifest. They know how to tell AD/HD from other disorders that mimic the symptoms of AD/HD. They know when it is too early to diagnose and when it is too late. An expert professional provides the best opportunity to obtain an accurate evaluation.

Referrals from others are the best way to find an expert. Seek out agencies and professionals that have special knowledge about AD/HD. Ask people you know for a recommendation. Your child's teacher, principal, and pediatrician are likely good sources for recommendations. Parents with children already diagnosed with AD/HD are usually excellent resources for referrals. Children and Adults with Attention-Deficit/Hyperactivity Disorder (CHADD), a national organization, can lead you to experts in AD/HD as well.

What type of doctor should evaluate my child?

There are varieties of professionals who are qualified to evaluate children for AD/HD. The most important thing about who you choose is not so much what their degree is, but rather that they have ample experience evaluating children for AD/HD.

Professionals who evaluate for AD/HD are:

- Pediatricians
- Developmental pediatricians
- Psychiatrists
- Pediatric neurologists
- Clinical psychologists
- Pediatric neuropsychologists
- Educational psychologists

While every professional will use the criteria listed in the mental health professionals' book of disorders, *Diagnostic and Statistical Manual of Mental Disorders IV-TR*, (DSM-IV-TR), each will have their own tools and procedures and each will have their own threshold for what level of symptoms they think meets criteria for the diagnosis.

There are some pros and cons in selecting which type of evaluator will assess your child. Pediatricians tend to have limited time. However, your pediatrician likely knows your child quite well and has a long-standing history of observing him. Psychiatrists, neurologists, and developmental pediatricians will all likely perform a longer evaluation, but the only form of intervention they have to offer is medication. Pediatric neuropsychologists and educational psychologists provide testing, but typically do not offer treatment. Clinical psychologists, many of whom can provide testing if necessary, can evaluate and provide treatment.

What should parents know about pediatricians?

Pediatricians are medical doctors who have a medical degree and have completed four years of medical school in addition to an internship and residency in their area of specialty. Pediatricians evaluate, diagnose, and treat childhood medical illnesses as well as monitor the development of children as they grow.

Parents often turn to their pediatrician when they notice their child is having behavioral difficulties. The advantage of seeing a pediatrician for behavioral problems is that they see hundreds of children and know what behavior is typical and what behavior is outside the norm. However, many parents seeking an evaluation for AD/HD have been disappointed in the evaluation they received from their pediatrician, usually consisting of a questionnaire they complete, a brief interview, and then a prescription, all within a fifteen- to twenty-minute period.

While many pediatricians are skilled in evaluating AD/HD, most of them structure their practice for short visits with an eye toward quick evaluation and quick treatment decisions. Pediatric practices are usually not designed for the lengthy interviews necessary to evaluate AD/HD. Parents can be disappointed when the only help they get is a prescription. However, a knowledgeable pediatrician follows the guidelines set by the American Academy of Pediatrics and will refer parents to a psychologist for behavioral treatment.

What should parents know about developmental pediatricians?

A developmental pediatrician is a medical doctor with a specialty in evaluating abnormalities in development and behavior in infants, toddlers, and children. These pediatricians are specialists in assessing a child's cognitive, social, behavioral, and physical development. Unlike a general pediatrician who primarily treats medical conditions in children, these specialists focus on the abnormal medical, psychological, neurological, genetic, behavioral, and developmental disorders of childhood.

Developmental pediatricians perform a physical examination, looking for medical causes of problems. They evaluate physical growth, motor development, and nutritional needs. They are skilled in screening for cognitive and speech and language delays. They also assess social and emotional development, along with adaptive development. A typical initial evaluation with a developmental pediatrician is comprehensive and lengthy and it is not uncommon for the appointment to last two hours or more.

For the AD/HD child, a developmental pediatrician can provide medication monitoring. However, because they are experts in the complete development of children, they take a team approach to the child, will typically advise parents to seek additional treatment with other professionals, and can usually provide recommendations.

What should parents know about child psychiatrists?

A child psychiatrist is a medical doctor who specializes in the evaluation and treatment of childhood mental disorders. Psychiatrists generally allow for at least a one-hour interview in their evaluation, with an eye toward the diagnosis and determination of medication needs. Most psychiatrists use medication as their sole form of treatment and do not provide psychotherapy or behavioral treatment. Some psychiatrists, however, will educate parents regarding the need for psychological and behavioral treatment.

Perhaps the most common disappointment experienced by parents when seeing a psychiatrist is their expectation that the psychiatrist will provide psychotherapy. Parents may feel rushed when the psychiatrist focuses the follow-up interviews on medication effectiveness and side effects. It is important for you to understand that a psychiatrist's job is to monitor the medication, not to provide psychotherapy or behavioral intervention. A psychiatrist will generally schedule a follow-up appointment within the first month. Once the medication is stable, most psychiatrists will have follow-up appointments every three to six months. While this is typical practice, recent research has shown that children who had monthly follow-up visits with the psychiatrist showed much greater improvement than those who saw their psychiatrist less frequently.

What should parents know about pediatric neurologists?

A pediatric neurologist is a physician who diagnoses and treats disorders of the nervous system in children. This includes diseases of the brain, spinal cord, nerves, and muscles. A pediatric neurologist may serve as a consultant to other physicians as well as provide long-term care to patients with chronic neurological disorders. They are the appropriate choice of physicians when tics or Tourette's syndrome is suspected in AD/HD children.

Parents seek a neurologist to be sure there are no neurological disorders present in their AD/HD child. Neurologists perform tests of nerve functioning by having the child engage in specific tasks. If brain or central nervous system dysfunction is suspected, the neurologist may suggest an EEG, CT, MRI, or other scans of the brain. These tests are not necessary in an evaluation for AD/HD and cannot determine the presence or absence of AD/HD, but they may be necessary to evaluate other nervous system disorders.

Once the child is given a clean bill of nervous system health, they generally do not see the neurologist again. If, however, the neurologist is selected by the parents to monitor the child's medication, then follow-up visits will be scheduled. Neurologists will likely be able to provide parents with a referral for psychological and behavioral treatment.

What should parents know about clinical psychologists?

Clinical psychologists have a PhD or PsyD, typically in clinical or counseling psychology. They provide evaluation, testing, and treatment.

Evaluation by a clinical psychologist will focus on determining the cause of the symptoms displayed. At least one hour is scheduled for the evaluation. This includes a history, a review of the child's report cards and academic achievement tests, observation of the child, behavioral analysis, and an interview of the parents and child.

The clinical psychologist may or may not use testing as part of the diagnostic procedure. Testing, although providing useful information, does not definitively tell if your child has AD/HD. Instead, the test results will be used by the psychologist as one piece of their evaluation.

Treatment provided by clinical psychologists includes various forms of psychotherapy. This includes individual, group, family, and couples treatment. Clinical psychologists who specialize in AD/HD are generally specialists in behavior modification and thus can provide parent education and training. A psychologist may offer all the necessary forms of treatment in his or her practice or be able to provide referrals to the other types of specialists.

Prescribing medication is not part of a psychologist's training and licensure in all but a few states and thus psychologists are generally prepared to provide referrals to MDs for medication.

What should parents know about pediatric neuropsychologists?

A pediatric neuropsychologist has a PhD, usually in clinical or counseling psychology, with post-doctoral specialty training in neuropsychology. These specialists study the individual functions of the brain and are able to evaluate a child's abilities in highly specific skills. For example, they not only evaluate a child's memory functioning, but can also assess their memory for visual, auditory, immediate, short-term and long-term abilities. Testing includes paper and pencil tests, oral tests, and tests requiring the manipulation of objects.

Neuropsychologists generally do not provide treatment for AD/HD, but instead offer specific recommendations based upon their test results. Recommendations are generally in the form of interventions to be carried out in school and during homework. Knowing a child's cognitive functions in specific detail can be very helpful in designing an educational program. Teachers and tutors can create lessons geared toward the child's specific strengths and weaknesses.

While a neuropsychological evaluation can provide detail about specific cognitive functions, it can be very expensive—costing $2000 or more. This type of in-depth testing is usually not necessary to make a diagnosis of AD/HD. Questions that are more specific are usually posed when a child is referred for neuropsychological testing, such as the suspicion of a learning disability, processing problems, and memory dysfunction.

What should parents know about educational psychologists?

Educational psychologists have a masters or doctorate degree in education, an MEd or EdD. They may evaluate and diagnose AD/HD, but more often, they usually focus on the evaluation and treatment of learning disorders and learning problems.

Educational psychologists perform evaluations through a variety of educational tests, including IQ and academic achievement tests. They are skilled at making very specific recommendations based upon those test results. Recommendations are designed for classroom and homework time. Educational psychologists are experts at applying those recommendations in a one-on-one setting with the student through educational therapy. They can also provide assistance in the design of a special education program.

Educational therapy is a process that combines an understanding of how learning takes place in the brain with knowledge of specialized teaching methods that help children learn. Educational psychologists can help children with AD/HD who do not have a learning disorder but still have difficulties with homework, organization, and planning of projects, books reports, and studying.

Due to budget and time constraints, the educational psychologist employed by your child's school will not provide the comprehensive testing and recommendations that a private practice educational psychologist can. Nor can they provide the educational therapy that a private practitioner can.

What should parents look for in choosing a doctor?

Not only is it difficult to choose which *type* of doctor to evaluate your child, it is equally as difficult to choose *who* that doctor will be. One of the most important factors in selecting your child's doctor is to find out whether or not he or she is able to view your child's entire functioning and develop a comprehensive treatment plan. Will the doctor take the time to review your child's records? Can the doctor provide referrals to address each of your child's needs? Will he work cooperatively with the other members of your child's treatment team, including the teacher?

The best way to choose a doctor is through a recommendation from others who know of the doctor's work and reputation. There are several ways to learn about your potential doctor before selecting her. Don't expect doctors to accept a phone call or to provide a free meeting in order for you to interview them. Instead, their receptionist or office manager is likely to answer many questions you have. You may also ask if they have a website and/or brochures that you can view. This will provide information about their degree, area of practice, specialties, philosophy of treatment, and interventions they are able to provide. Once you have found a doctor that you think might be right for your child, you are ready to schedule an appointment. Ask for an evaluation to determine if your child has ADD or ADHD.

What medical tests are used to diagnose AD/HD?

There are no medical tests to determine if ADD or ADHD exists. Unlike a medical condition where a blood, urine, x-ray, or brainwave test provides exact answers, AD/HD has no definitive test.

When parents are advised that they should have their child "tested" for AD/HD, what they really are being told is they need to have their child evaluated. Testing refers to specific laboratory exams that give exact answers to whether or not something exists, such as a bladder infection or a broken bone. Despite some physicians using such medical techniques as an EEG or QEEG (Electroencephalogram and Quantitative Electroencephalogram), no medical test currently exists that can determine if someone has AD/HD. Such procedures are not supported by the vast majority of medical practitioners or the American Pediatric Association.

Parents must be informed so that they do not waste time, effort, money, and hope on tests that cannot provide a diagnosis. Instead, parents should seek an experienced evaluator who informs them that the diagnosis is based upon the evaluator's clinical judgment rather than medical tests. Evaluators tend to review a variety of information such as parent and teacher reports, as well as observation of the child to make their determination.

What psychological or educational tests are used to diagnose AD/HD?

There are no psychological or educational tests that will definitively determine if a child has AD/HD. Testing is rarely done for diagnosing ADHD, as the hyperactive symptoms are readily observed. However, if ADD is in question and cannot be confidently diagnosed based upon history, observation, record review, and behavioral analysis, then educational testing can be helpful as part of the diagnostic evaluation.

Unlike the annual academic achievement testing conducted each year at school, educational testing must be administered face-to-face by either a clinical or an educational psychologist. The testing will generally include an IQ test and an academic achievement battery. In addition to seeing how the child's scores compare to (those of other children her age), the psychologist is able to closely observe the child's behavior during the several hours of test administration.

The evaluator will observe how the child approaches tasks that are similar to school and homework. They will observe the child's ability to sit still while working, pay attention, stick to tasks (some of which may be boring), tolerate frustration, ignore distractions, stay motivated, and remain focused.

Do children behave differently in a one-on-one testing situation?

When testing is introduced into the diagnostic evaluation, you may be concerned that the results are distorted because of the one-on-one interaction. Typically, children do better in a one-on-one situation when compared to the classroom or during homework. This is actually an asset to the diagnostic evaluation. The benefit provided by one-on-one testing is the psychologist's ability to measure the child's true abilities. Without the distractions of the classroom, and with the added novelty of meeting with the psychologist, children generally enjoy the testing and try hard to please the evaluator. This allows the psychologist to measure what the child truly knows, even if his knowledge is not reflected in his work or on his report cards.

The second benefit of one-on-one testing is that because it takes four to eight hours to complete, the psychologist is usually able to observe the child in several different sessions. Once the novelty wears off and the desire to please becomes hard to sustain, the child eventually displays his typical behavior. Even under the ideal situation of a quiet office and one-on-one attention, children with AD/HD can't help but display their symptoms.

If I have my child tested, what tests should be used?

Before selecting which tests will be administered, a psychologist must have specific questions that the tests will provide answers to. The most common reason to use testing in an evaluation for AD/HD is to determine if a learning disorder is present. To answer this question, the evaluator will administer a standardized IQ test; the most commonly used being the Wechsler tests, of which there is a preschool, elementary/middle school, and high school/adult version. These tests are not the same as paper and pencil IQ tests sold at bookstores and on the Internet. These are the gold standard for accurate IQ testing and occur face-to-face.

A learning disorder evaluation will also include an academic achievement test battery. These are also administered face-to-face to the child by the psychologist. Commonly used tests include Woodcock Johnson III, Kaufman, and the Peabody Individual Achievement Test.

A minimum test battery should include IQ and academic achievement testing. Numerous additional tests may be administered, each for a specific purpose. Tests for specific cognitive functions may be administered in order to determine the areas of strength and weakness in cognitive functioning.

What use do I make out of the test results?

In order to make the time, effort, and expense of testing worthwhile, the psychologist must be able to interpret the meaning of the results and provide specific recommendations. It is not uncommon to spend $2,000 for a test battery and come to the end of a twenty-page report only to read the conclusion that your child has trouble concentrating, a fact you already knew!

Before agreeing to a test battery, it is acceptable to ask to read either a description of what the psychologist will be looking for in the testing and/or a sample report (with names removed for privacy). By reading a sample report, you will be able to determine if the psychologist is going to be able to provide results that you can understand and clear recommendations about what to do. After all, "what to do next" is one of the main reasons to test. Do not agree to testing, unless the psychologist will prepare a written report of the test results, interpretation, and recommendations.

Once you have the test report, provide a copy to each professional working with your child. Schedule a meeting with each professional to discuss the results and what interventions they suggest.

What information can an IQ test provide?

The majority of parents believe their child is smart or bright. While we all want to think our children are intelligent, the truth is that 82 percent of us are average. Only 9 percent of us are truly intellectually bright and 9 percent of us are well below average. So, if most of us are average, then why bother to take a test to find that out?

IQ testing tells us how intellectually *capable* we are. It tells us who is truly gifted, who may need a slower-paced class, and who can be expected to succeed in the average classroom. Academic placement decisions are easier to make and expectations are easier to set when we know a child's IQ. A child with a low average IQ who has parents who insist on straight A's is likely to encounter stress, feelings of failure, and low self-esteem.

IQ testing also tells us strengths and weaknesses across many areas. It tells us verbal abilities in comparison to visual-perceptual abilities. It provides information on long-term learning, immediate memory, social judgment, understanding cause and effect, and abstract thinking, among others.

What information can academic achievement tests provide?

Academic achievement testing measures what a child has learned over the past academic year. Test scores will tell you what grade level and age level of knowledge your child has achieved in a wide variety of academic skills and subjects. It is most commonly used to help determine if your child has a learning disorder. If your child's academic achievement level is significantly below his IQ level, then a learning disorder is likely present.

Even without the presence of a learning disorder, academic achievement testing provides rich information about what a child has learned and whether or not he has reached grade level.

Academic achievement testing is very helpful in making decisions about a child's school placement and medication. Report cards reflect how a child has performed, not what they have actually learned. Academic achievement testing will measure what grade level a child has achieved over the year, independent of his report card. A child can have very low grades, rarely do his homework, and have a lot of behavior problems, but nonetheless learn during the school year. Parents can rest easier knowing that despite a poor report card, the child has learned what he was supposed to learn.

What information can personality testing provide?

Personality testing, or psychological testing as it is called, provides a wealth of information about a child's personality style. It offers a look inside the child's emotional mind, showing parts of his world that cannot easily be observed. Interpersonal style, coping skills, world outlook, problem solving style, mood, and self-esteem can be determined by personality test results. These aspects of the AD/HD child are often overlooked in the effort to get them to do their homework, settle down, pay attention, and cooperate. The subtle forms of anxiety and depression that AD/HD children often have are not easily observed, yet can readily be discovered during psychological testing.

This type of testing involves activities that most children find enjoyable, such as drawing pictures, telling stories about pictures, and completing sentences. As children get older, they are able to take self-report tests where they can answer questions about their feelings and behavior. Psychological testing should include several tests to obtain a comprehensive picture. Results can be immensely helpful for the psychotherapist working with your child in providing an in-depth picture of your child's internal world. Interventions can be designed specifically for your child based upon the test results.

How often should testing be done?
Unlike certain medical tests that have a standard time frame to repeat, there is no set schedule of when IQ, academic achievement, or neuropsychological testing should be done. Once a test battery is completed, the benefit of re-administering the tests is to measure progress. Most psychologists would say that at least one year should pass before testing is repeated. This may even be too soon; as progress with learning disorders and AD/HD is slow, and measurable success may not show up after one year. Two to three years is a more reasonable period that allows the child to benefit from the academic, behavioral, and psychological interventions.

There can be exceptions to this general recommendation. If testing is to be done more frequently, there should be a specific purpose and a plan for modifying interventions based upon the results. Re-testing should involve a comparison of both sets of test data. Having the same psychologist administer the re-testing has the advantage of their experience with, and prior knowledge of, the child. If you choose a different psychologist for a re-test, be sure they are provided with the previous test data and written report so they may do an accurate comparison.

What information can school achievement tests provide?

Each year, schools administer standardized academic achievement tests in a paper and pencil format that an entire class takes at the same time. Commonly used tests include Stanford Achievement Test, Iowa Test of Basic Skills, Scholastic Aptitude Test, Comprehensive Test of Basic Skills, and California Achievement Test,. These tests provide a measure of what the child has learned in school during the past year in various academic areas. They are not a substitute for the individually administered academic achievement tests, but are a useful measure of how the child is progressing from year to year in the basic subject areas.

It is important to bring all of your child's annual academic achievement test scores to an evaluator. This will help determine if testing for a learning disorder is necessary. It will also help in recommendations for academic placement. It is not unusual to have a child with AD/HD be near failing in school, but have annual achievement test scores in the 90th percentile. Nor is it unusual for a child to have very high scores one year, extremely low the following year, and average the next. This is a potential sign of AD/HD and can be indicative of trouble sustaining the mental effort needed to perform well on these tests.

What information can report cards provide?

Report cards are often mistaken for a measure of the child's learning throughout the school year. However, these are more a measure of a child's performance, and only partially reflect his learning. Instead, academic achievement tests tell what a child has *learned*. Report cards largely tell how the child did in producing and completing work, being accurate in his answers, writing properly, and cooperating with the teacher, among other skills.

Children with AD/HD often have very poor report cards due to their difficulty producing the volume, neatness, and timeliness of work requested by teachers. Placing pressure on a child with AD/HD to earn high grades can lead to high frustration, feelings of failure, low self-esteem, a dislike for learning, resentment towards parents, and frequent family conflict over homework.

Society has placed an overemphasis on report cards. Reflect back on your own report cards, those of your spouse, friends, and family. How many of you achieved consistently high grades? How much is your life affected today by your fourth grade report card? Do you even remember your fourth grade report card? How many of you grew up to lead a nice, responsible, moral, ethical, and happy life despite not being an "A" student? Keep this in mind when setting expectations for your child's grades.

Can a diagnosis be made from a behavior checklist?

Behavior checklists are standardized questionnaires that list a wide variety of behaviors that children engage in. Many parents are alarmed when their doctor relies on a behavior checklist in making the diagnosis of AD/HD. While this should not be the sole source of information, the behavior checklist is a very useful diagnostic tool. While it is quick for parents to fill out and quick for doctors to score and interpret, decades of research have gone on behind the scenes to develop these checklists and make them useful.

Here's how they work. Researchers provide a lengthy list of behaviors that children engage in. They find very large groups of parents to complete the questionnaires. By having thousands of parents who have children free of problems complete the questionnaire, the researchers are able to see what so called "normal" children look like in terms of mood and behavior. By having thousands of parents whose children have disorders complete the checklist, they are able to see how children with a variety of problems appear on the checklist. Your child's test scores are examined to see if he more closely matches the "normal" group or the depressed, anxious, hyperactive, inattentive, aggressive, socially problematic, or other disordered group.

Can a diagnosis of AD/HD be made from a computerized test?

No test can make a diagnosis of AD/HD—including computerized tests. If a computerized test is given, it should be used only as an additional supplementary tool, not the sole or primary source of diagnosis. Unfortunately, there are evaluators who rely solely or heavily on computerized testing to prove that a child has AD/HD.

Computerized testing can be very expensive—in the hundreds of dollars. The results tell you how well your child attended to the test and how well he resisted impulsive responses. The theory is that children with AD/HD will do poorly because they will fail to pay sufficient attention and they will be unable to resist the impulse to respond before carefully considering their answers.

AD/HD children do indeed perform poorly on these types of tests. Is this worth the hundreds of dollars that parents pay? Most professionals would say no. Parents already know the child has attention problems, hence the reason for the evaluation. Since a computerized test is not a definitive diagnostic tool and it does not provide new information about the child, it hardly warrants the expense.

What information should I tell the doctor?

Preparing for an evaluation or meeting with a new doctor is very important. Pediatricians are especially limited on their time, with the average office visit lasting only ten minutes. Psychologists and psychiatrists typically have an average visit of one hour. There is a lot of information to cover in ten to sixty minutes. Organization and preparation can help ensure a thorough evaluation.

Many evaluators have lengthy questionnaires for parents to fill out before the visit. While this exhausts some parents, it can save time and allows the doctor to focus her interview on the most relevant questions. Be sure to answer honestly, even if you feel embarrassed. Your doctor can only do her job with accurate information.

Prepare ahead of time and gather the necessary information to answer questions about your child's family history. Background about siblings, parents, grandparents, and aunts and uncles can be useful in the following categories:

- Mental health history
- History of ADD/ADHD/ODD/CD/Antisocial Personality Disorder
- Substance abuse history
- Criminal history
- School and learning history
- Behavior problems
- Mood and/or behavior medication history
- Suicide history
- Highest grade completed
- Divorce and step-family constellation
- Trauma History

What records should I give to the doctor?

Your child's records are an essential piece of the information needed to perform a diagnostic evaluation. AD/HD in particular is a disorder that relies heavily on a thorough recording of history. Without records, the evaluator can rely only on what you tell him and what he observes in his office.

The following records are important for your doctor to consider in the diagnostic evaluation:

- Report cards
- Annual academic achievement test scores
- Individual education plans
- Notes sent home from school
- Educational testing reports
- Personality testing reports
- AD/HD prior evaluation results

The easier you make it for your doctor to review the records, the more likely it is that he will take the time to read them. Prepare a copy of all the records for the doctor to keep in his file. Call the doctor's office and ask if you may send the records before the evaluation in case doctor has time to review them before your visit. Organize your records by category and place them in order from oldest to most recent, this way the doctor can see the changes in your child from year to year by simply turning to the next page.

What questions will the doctor ask me about my child?

Much of the information your doctor needs will be contained in the records you send or bring with you, the behavior checklist you complete, and the history questionnaire you fill out. Combined, these help your doctor narrow down the questions she will ask you. You can assist your doctor by being an accurate and concise reporter. Bring a list of the behaviors you observe in your child and be sure to tell the doctor about them. Be prepared to provide information regarding how well your child is able to:

- Sit still
- Wait his turn
- Complete class work
- Keep track of her belongings
- Complete homework in a timely fashion
- Return homework to the teacher
- Complete book reports and projects
- Get ready for school
- Complete chores
- Follow instructions
- Complete requests without repeated reminders or nagging

- Get along with peers
- Cooperate with rules
- Make and keep friends
- Manage his anger
- Remember rules, items, and instructions
- Play quietly
- Join a conversation or game
- Delay gratification
- Think before she acts
- Keep belongings organized
- Show emotional maturity
- Be aware of his behavior
- Manage her feelings
- Avoid minor distractions

What if the evaluation is inconclusive?

It is not uncommon to have a diagnostic evaluation be inconclusive. Because AD/HD is based on clinical judgment, there are cases where one doctor will determine the disorder is present but another doctor will say it is not. Your child may be too young to determine if the disorder is fully present, or the symptoms may not be severe enough to warrant the diagnosis. Doctors differ on where they draw the line for diagnosing. This is not surprising and merely highlights the somewhat subjective nature of diagnosing this disorder.

If your child's evaluation is inconclusive, there are several options to consider. You may opt to obtain a second opinion with the same type of doctor who performed the first evaluation, thus having two opinions from two different psychologists. Alternatively, you may seek a different category of specialist, thus having an opinion, for example, from one psychologist and one psychiatrist. Educational or neuropsychological testing may provide the additional information necessary to render a diagnosis. Finally, as many parents do, you can simply choose to have your child treated for the various problems he exhibits and not be concerned about the actual diagnosis.

Chapter 3

COEXISTING DISORDERS

- Is it really AD/HD or is it something else?
- How many AD/HD children have a second disorder?
- What is Oppositional Defiant Disorder?
- What should parents know about ODD?
- What is Conduct Disorder?
- What should parents know about Conduct Disorder?
- What is Asperger's Disorder?
- What should parents know about Asperger's Disorder?
- What is a learning disorder?
- What should parents know about learning disorders?
- What is Tourette's syndrome?
- What should parents know about Tourette's syndrome?
- What is childhood depression?
- What should parents know about childhood depression?
- What is childhood anxiety?
- What should parents know about childhood anxiety?
- What is Obsessive-Compulsive Disorder?
- What should parents know about Obsessive-Compulsive Disorder?
- What is Bipolar Disorder?
- What should parents know about Bipolar Disorder?
- What is Developmental Coordination Disorder?
- What should parents know about Developmental Coordination Disorder?
- What is Enuresis and Encopresis?
- What should parents know about Enuresis and Encopresis ?

Is it really AD/HD or is it something else?

With the exception of Oppositional Defiant Disorder, other conditions are not often mistaken for ADHD. However, many disorders
and situational problems of childhood can look like ADD. When a
child is struggling with school and homework, one of the first things
considered is ADD. If you run down the checklist of symptoms of
ADD, the child can quickly, but perhaps erroneously, be diagnosed
with ADD.

When children are struggling with learning, social, family, or
emotional issues, it usually affects their school and homework.
Learning disorders, divorce, trauma, and social rejection are just a
few of the things that can cause symptoms similar to ADD.
Children may daydream as a means to escape negative feelings and
have trouble mustering up enough effort to do their homework.
They are not always able to tell teachers and parents that they are
upset and having trouble concentrating or are unable to learn.
Instead, their distress manifests in their behavior and school
performance.

Since many childhood problems can look like the symptoms of
ADD, it is very important that a child who appears to have ADD be
evaluated for other disorders.

How many children with AD/HD have a second disorder?

As if AD/HD were not enough for one child and one family to cope
with; unfortunately, AD/HD rarely exists by itself. More children
than not have at least one other disorder. It is estimated that approximately two thirds of children with AD/HD have at least one other
mental disorder and as many as 10 percent have three or more disorders. Multiple disorders are the norm rather than the exception.
The coexisting disorder has a significant influence on how AD/HD

symptoms are manifested and how they affect mood, behavior, and academic functioning. Treatment will vary depending on the secondary disorder.

The most common coexisting disorder is Oppositional Defiant Disorder, with approximately one third of those with AD/HD having this disruptive behavior disorder. Twenty-five to 40 percent of children with ODD go on to develop Conduct Disorder. Depression, anxiety, tic disorder, and Tourette's are other common coexisting disorders. Depression is present in 10 to 30 percent of children diagnosed with AD/HD. Anxiety disorders exist in approximately 25 to 30 percent of children with AD/HD. This includes generalized anxiety, phobias, obsessive-compulsive disorder, and separation anxiety disorder.

While only 20 to 30 percent of children with AD/HD have a diagnosable learning disorder, at least 60 percent have learning problems. The breakdown of coexisting disorders looks something like this:

- Second disorder: 66 percent
- Learning problems: 60 percent
- Oppositional Defiant Disorder: 33 percent
- Anxiety Disorder: 25 to 30 percent
- Conduct Disorder: 25 percent
- Depression: 10 to 30 percent
- Obsessive-Compulsive Disorder: 10 to 17 percent
- Three or more disorders: 10 percent
- Learning disorders: 10 percent
- Tourette's: 7 percent

What is Oppositional Defiant Disorder?

Oppositional Defiant Disorder (ODD) is a recurrent pattern of defiant, disobedient, oppositional, negative, and hostile behavior toward adults. Children with ODD have four or more of the following symptoms:

- Spiteful or vindictive
- Loses temper
- Angry and resentful
- Argues with adults
- Touchy or easily annoyed
- Actively defies or refuses to comply with adults' requests or rules
- Blames others for his or her mistakes or misbehavior
- Deliberately annoys people

Symptoms must be present for at least six months and occur more frequently than is typical for age and developmental level. Some oppositional behavior is expected in toddler and preschool children as a normal part of development. Therefore, ODD is only diagnosed in very young children if the pattern of behavior is significantly more frequent and intense when compared to others the same age. The same is expected of teens who typically become a bit more defiant as they become independent from their parents. However, when a teen has a frequent and intense pattern of defiance, she may have ODD. These symptoms usually appear at home. In environments outside the home, such as school, sports, or social activities, the symptoms may not appear and the ODD child can be viewed by others as pleasant.

What should parents know about ODD?

The ODD child is a very difficult child to raise, refusing to comply with even the most basic request. They want their way and few things will stop them from getting it. They live by the philosophy of "you're not the boss of me!" Constant battles result in a cycle of negativity between the parent and the child and they tend to bring out the worst in one another.

Two to 16 percent of children have ODD, yet for those with AD/HD, this number rises dramatically to approximately one third. This is the most common combination of disorders for AD/HD children, and the most difficult. ODD children begin as very demanding and willful toddlers and continue to become increasingly stubborn, oppositional, and angry with each passing year. ODD usually develops before eight years of age.

Medication is not effective for ODD. Parents must learn behavior modification skills and commit to consistent parenting. Children with AD/HD coexisting with ODD have poorer outcomes than children with just AD/HD. In a large number of children, ODD develops into Conduct Disorder, a more serious behavior disorder. The good news is that ODD can be overcome with long-term treatment.

What is Conduct Disorder?

Conduct Disorder (CD) is a persistent pattern of behavior where rules and rights of others are violated. Children with CD have at least three of the following symptoms:

- Bullying, threatening, or intimidating others
- Starting physical fights
- Use of a weapon
- Physical cruelty to people

- Physical cruelty to animals
- Stolen while confronting a victim
- Forced someone into sexual activity
- Deliberately engaged in setting fires to cause serious damage
- Deliberately destroyed others' property
- Broken into someone's car, building, or home
- Lies or cons others to gain something or avoid an obligation
- Stolen without confronting a victim, e.g. shoplifting
- Stays out at night despite parental rules, starting before age thirteen
- Runs away from home overnight
- Truant from school, beginning before age thirteen

Less serious symptoms of CD can begin in early elementary school and advance as the child matures and expands his repertoire of antisocial behaviors. These children and adolescents are aggressive toward others, deceitful, destructive of others' property, and repeatedly violate rules. CD is seen more in males than females. The earlier the symptoms begin, the more serious the disorder and the greater risk the child has to develop Antisocial Personality Disorder.

What should parents know about Conduct Disorder?

Conduct Disorder is a serious behavior disorder. AD/HD is common in children with Conduct Disorder, with about 25 percent having both disorders. Symptoms may start as early as five or six years old, but typically start in later childhood and early adolescence. Onset usually starts with less severe behaviors in the younger years, such as lying, stealing, and physical fights, and gradually increases to more severe behaviors as the child gets older. The earlier the onset, the worse the prognosis is.

Males are much more likely to have Conduct Disorder than females. Males have a rate of Conduct Disorder from 6 to 16 percent, whereas female rates range from 2 to 9 percent. Males tend to engage in more fighting, stealing, vandalism, and behavior problems at school. Females are more prone to lie, be truant, and run away from home.

Conduct Disorder is associated with early onset of sexual behavior, drinking, smoking, drug use, and reckless and risk-taking acts. Children with this disorder are commonly suspended or expelled from school. Academic achievement is often low. Many adolescents grow out of the disorder; however, a large number go on to develop Antisocial Personality Disorder, a very serious problem of antisocial behavior in adults.

What is Asperger's Disorder?

Asperger's is a disorder of severe and persistent problems with social interaction and restricted patterns of interests, activities, and behavior. Children with Asperger's have at least two of the following impairments in social interaction and at least one impairment in behavior:

- Lack of social or emotional reciprocity
- Marked impairment in non-verbal behavior
- Lack of spontaneous seeking of sharing interests and pleasure with others
- Failure to develop appropriate peer relationships
- Preoccupied with restricted patterns of interest
- Preoccupied with parts of objects
- Inflexible adherence to rituals
- Repetitive motor movements

Children with Asperger's are average or bright intellectually, but are perceived by others as rather odd socially. Symptoms may not become apparent until they enter school and have difficulties making friends. These children are self-focused and show little awareness or interest in others except for having an audience to talk to about their very specific and narrow interests. They have trouble with eye contact, body language, and the give and take of conversations and relationships. They can be extremely interested in one or two subjects and focus most talking and activities around that topic. They can be insistent that they be allowed to engage in behaviors that have no usefulness.

What should parents know about Asperger's Disorder?

Asperger's Disorder is a relatively new disorder, first listed in the *DSM-IV* in 1994. Consequently, little is known about its causes, course, and treatment. It is not a clearly defined and easily made diagnosis. It is more common in males. Symptoms often surface in school when the social difficulties become apparent by peer rejection. This disorder is thought to last throughout life with no cure. Some researchers view Asperger's as a milder form of autism.

These children's primary deficit is in social interactions and relationships. Children with Asperger's have an inability to understand what is going on in the minds of others. They lack empathy and are unable to understand how other people feel and how they might react to the Asperger's child's words and behavior. They do not understand how to behave toward others. They miss out on nonverbal cues, not understanding facial expressions, gestures, and body language.

They fail to consider what others might need and instead focus on their immediate thoughts, feelings, and desires. They dominate conversations and become frustrated when others interrupt them or try to change the subject. They cannot shift gears in conversations or activities without upset. Combined with AD/HD, they have a tremendous struggle for social success.

What is a learning disorder?

Learning disorders occur when a child's academic achievement in a specific subject is significantly below what would be expected for their age, school experience, and intellectual ability. Learning disorders can occur in reading, mathematics, and writing, with reading accounting for about 80 percent.

To determine if a child has a learning disorder, she must undergo standardized academic achievement testing to assess what age level and grade level of learning she has achieved. An IQ test must also be given in order to assess the child's intellectual capabilities. Generally, if the child has a discrepancy of more than two standard deviations difference between academic achievement and IQ, a learning disorder is diagnosed.

There may be underlying problems in processing information that precede or are associated with a learning disorder. Children with a learning disorder may have deficits in specific cognitive functions such as memory, auditory processing, visual processing, and attention, among others.

Reading Disorders, which have also been called "dyslexia," manifest in impairments of reading accuracy, speed, or comprehension. Mathematics Disorders are displayed by impairment in mathematical calculation or mathematical reasoning. Written Expression Disorder is manifested by impairment in the ability to compose written text due to trouble with punctuation, grammar, organization, spelling, and excessively poor handwriting.

What should parents know about learning disorders?

Learning disorders are commonly mistaken for AD/HD. When children have trouble learning, they may show symptoms making them appear to have AD/HD. Without proper evaluation, learning disorders can easily be overlooked and/or misdiagnosed as AD/HD. Approximately 10 percent of children with AD/HD also have a learning disorder.

A review of the child's report cards and annual academic achievement test scores are a good first step in discovering if a learning disorder exists. A child who has one or more academic areas significantly below his other areas may have a learning disorder. Learning disorders are present in all levels of intelligence. A child with a learning disorder may be gifted, average, or even below average.

Learning disorders are treated with special education and educational therapy. Some children with a learning disorder remain in the regular or "mainstream" classroom full time. Others stay mainstreamed, but have "resource" services for one or more hours per week where they are placed with a special education teacher who helps them learn techniques to compensate for their specific learning disorder. Children with more severe learning disorders may be placed in a full-time special education classroom or go to a private school that specializes in learning disorders.

What is Tourette's syndrome?

Tourette's is a disorder of multiple tics, including motor and vocal tics that are present for more than one year. A tic is a sudden, rapid, involuntary, and recurrent stereotyped movement or vocalization. Tics are experienced as being irresistible, but can be suppressed for varying lengths of time. Tics can be suppressed during periods of interesting activities. Alternatively, they can be increased by stress. Examples of simple motor tics include eye blinking, facial grimacing, coughing, shoulder shrugging, and neck jerking. Complex motor tics may include facial gestures, touching, and smelling an object. Simple vocal tics may include sniffing, snorting, barking, throat clearing, and grunting. Complex vocal tics include repeating words or phrases out of context, swearing, and repeating the last word or phrase heard.

The frequency and types of tics present in Tourette's change over time. Most often, Tourette's begins with a simple tic of eye blinking. Tics may disappear for periods of time, leading one to think it has disappeared. The same tic may return or new types of tics may take its place.

Tourette's most commonly starts in childhood and is strongly associated with hyperactivity, distractibility, and impulsivity. It can be exacerbated by central nervous system stimulant medication that is commonly given for AD/HD.

What should parents know about Tourette's syndrome?

Tourette's syndrome is seen in approximately four to five individuals per 10,000. It is one-and-a-half to three times more common in males than females. It can start as early as two years old, but more commonly starts in childhood or adolescence. Once the tics surface, they usually last a lifetime. It is most often a genetic disorder, with only 10 percent of those afflicted having the non-genetic type.

If a child has Tourette's, he likely has ADHD, as 60 percent of children with Tourette's also have ADHD. Fortunately, the reverse is not true; only 7 percent of children with ADHD have Tourette's. Depression, anxiety, low self-esteem, and embarrassment are also experienced by children with Tourette's. School functioning can also be impaired by the obsessions and compulsions that often coexist with Tourette's.

There is a link between tics and stimulant medication. While there is debate as to whether or not tics can be caused by stimulants, or if they merely bring about tics that would have surfaced anyway, most physicians recommend that stimulant medication be stopped altogether at the first sign of tics.

While neuroleptic medication is the only form of treatment for tics, most physicians avoid prescribing this major tranquilizing drug, preferring instead to let the tics occur naturally.

What is childhood depression?

Children are usually unaware of what depression is and unlikely to verbalize it. Instead, they show their depression in complaints of not feeling well, irritable moods, and social withdrawal. Teens are more aware of their mood and therefore may be more vocal about their depression. Symptoms of depression include:

- Depressed or irritable mood
- Decreased interest or pleasure in activities
- Changes in weight or appetite
- Insomnia or excessive sleeping
- Physical agitation or retardation
- Fatigue or loss of energy

- Feelings of worthlessness or guilt
- Decreased concentration
- Thoughts of death or suicide

Major Depressive Episodes occur abruptly and cause dramatic change in normal functioning. The child or teen may cry a lot, be very irritable, have little motivation to do anything, and find little pleasure in activities he previously enjoyed. Sleep and appetite changes occur, as do changes in schoolwork. Self-esteem can become very low and children and teens may talk negatively about themselves.

Dysthymic Disorder is a chronic depression that slowly emerges and lasts for at least one year. Irritable and cranky moods exist alongside negative self-esteem and a pessimistic view on life. The depressed mood comes and goes, with happiness lasting no longer than two months.

What should parents know about childhood depression?

Ten to 30 percent of children with AD/HD are thought to have depression. For these children the depression may not be obvious. Rather than an abrupt change from a usually happy mood to a sad mood, children with AD/HD have a more subtle and slowly emerging onset of depression. Their sadness stems from a daily life of not fitting in at school, being teased and rejected by their peers, annoying their classmates and teachers, failing to meet academic standards, and upsetting their parents with their behavior. These struggles can lead some children with AD/HD to have low self-esteem and periods of unhappiness. Adding to their sadness may be a sense of hopelessness that comes from their inability to control their AD/HD symptoms.

As the children grow from year to year, they become more aware of their differences from others and their inability to fit in, leading to increased risk for depression as they move through childhood to adolescence. Suicidal ideation is not uncommon and must be treated seriously and not regarded as an attempt for attention.

Individual psychotherapy, group psychotherapy, and medication can be very effective in treating childhood depression.

What is childhood anxiety?

Generalized Anxiety Disorder in children and teens is characterized by persistent and excessive worry that lasts for at least six months. Symptoms of anxiety include:

- Excessive anxiety and worry
- Difficulty controlling the worry
- Feeling restless or on edge
- Easily fatigued
- Difficulty concentrating
- Irritability
- Muscle tension
- Sleep disturbance

All children have worries from time to time, but children with Generalized Anxiety Disorder are excessively worried and the symptoms are significantly distressing and cause impairment in functioning. The most common worries for children are school or sports performance, and catastrophic events such as earthquakes. Anxious children tend to be perfectionists and may need excessive reassurance.

The worrying experienced by children with anxiety disorders can appear similar to symptoms of AD/HD. When children cannot get their mind off their worries, it is difficult for them to concentrate, pay attention, and focus on their school and homework.

More specific types of anxiety disorders in children and teens are usually more rapid in onset than Generalized Anxiety Disorder. Separation Anxiety Disorder occurs when children are excessively fearful of being away from their parent or caretaker. Specific Phobias are intense fears and avoidance of specific things, events, or places. School Phobia is a common Specific Phobia. Panic Disorder is characterized by abrupt episodes of intense fear that are accompanied by physical symptoms. Social Phobia includes excessive fear of social situations where the child or teen fears they will do something to embarrass themselves.

What should parents know about childhood anxiety?

About 25 to 30 percent of children with AD/HD experience anxiety. Unfortunately, children are usually not even aware of what anxiety is and are unable to tell parents what they are experiencing, therefore making it difficult for parents to know that their child is anxious. Anxiety in children can be more easily observed in their behavior than heard in their words.

Two hallmark indicators of anxiety are complaining and avoidance. Anxious children will complain of having headaches, stomachaches, and generally feeling ill despite being in good health. Some children may truly feel sick and even vomit from intense anxiety. It is not difficult for children to figure out that complaining about feeling sick is a good way to escape having to do things that make them nervous. Anxious children may also use tantrums, resistance, oppositionalism, and defiance to escape situations that cause them anxiety. These noncompliant symptoms can easily be mistaken for AD/HD, as they are the same behaviors displayed by AD/HD children trying to escape homework and chores.

Other symptoms of anxiety include irritable mood, fatigue, poor concentration, shyness, nail biting, thumb sucking, bed-wetting, day-time wetting, skin picking, insomnia, and nightmares. Such children may also be excessively shy and withdrawn and physically cling to parents.

While many children experience these symptoms at various points, anxious children experience them frequently and intensely. Children with AD/HD and coexisting anxiety can be expected to have a more dramatic presentation of some of their AD/HD symptoms, as there is a large overlap in the way the symptoms are displayed in both disorders.

What is Obsessive-Compulsive Disorder?

Obsessive-Compulsive Disorder (OCD) is marked by recurrent obsessions and compulsions that interfere with daily functioning and/or cause distresses. Obsessions are recurrent and persistent ideas, thoughts, impulses, or images that are intrusive and cause distress. The thoughts are unwanted and not within the child or teen's control and go excessively beyond normal worries. Compulsions are repetitive behaviors that serve the sole purpose of preventing or reducing anxiety. The child or teen feels driven to perform the behavior, sometimes to prevent a dreaded result, such as washing hands in order to prevent disease. Some obsessions include performing rigid or stereotyped behaviors that have no real function or connection to preventing the dreaded event.

Children may not be aware of their obsessions and compulsions and therefore may not report them to others. Teens are usually more aware and likely to report that both obsessions and compulsions are unwanted and that they have made unsuccessful attempts to suppress them.

Common obsessions include fears of contamination, a need to have things in exact order, and fears of having done a horrible deed. Common compulsions include hand washing, counting, putting things in order, checking that doors are locked, and having to perform tasks in a highly specific order.

What should parents know about Obsessive-Compulsive Disorder?

OCD coexists in approximately 10 to 17 percent of children with AD/HD. Symptoms of OCD can intensify the struggles that AD/HD children have to contend with. The AD/HD child with OCD can easily become overwhelmed trying to comply with requests, follow directions, and complete tasks in the midst of having thoughts he cannot get rid of and rituals he "must" do. Arguments with parents, frustration, and anger outbursts are not uncommon as the child simply cannot comply with requests to stop his compulsion. Already struggling to make friends, the AD/HD child with OCD may withdraw from socializing as a way to hide his compulsions from his peers and prevent being teased. Paying attention in class and to homework, already a challenge for the AD/HD child, is further compounded by the distraction of thoughts the child cannot make stop. His work may be interrupted by behaviors he "has to do."

Medication is the most effective treatment for OCD. Several types of antidepressants have been found to control the obsessions and compulsions. They have the added benefit of improving mood, which can in turn decrease some of the irritability seen in children with AD/HD. Psychotherapy can help with the related anxiety, embarrassment, and social difficulties that typically accompany OCD.

What is Bipolar Disorder?

Bipolar Disorder is characterized by alternating episodes of depression and mania or mixed mood states where both mania and depression rapidly cycle. These episodes cause unusual shifts in mood, energy, and behavior that interfere with normal, healthy functioning.

Bipolar disorder is difficult to diagnose, as it looks very different in children than it does in adults. Symptoms of mania and depression in children and adolescents manifest themselves through a variety of different behaviors. When manic, children and adolescents are more likely to be irritable and prone to destructive outbursts than to be elated or euphoric like adults with Bipolar Disorder. When depressed, there may be physical complaints such as headaches, muscle aches, stomachaches, or tiredness, frequent absences from school or poor performance in school, talk of or efforts to run away from home, irritability, complaining, unexplained crying, social isolation, poor communication, and sensitivity to rejection or failure. Other manifestations of manic and depressive states in teens may include alcohol or substance abuse, hyper-sexuality, and difficulty with friendships.

Existing evidence indicates that Bipolar Disorder beginning in childhood or early adolescence may be a different, possibly more severe form of the illness than older adolescent and adult onset Bipolar Disorder.

What should parents know about Bipolar Disorder?

Although once thought rare in children, approximately 7 percent of children seen at psychiatric facilities are diagnosed with Bipolar Disorder. One of the biggest challenges has been to differentiate children with manic symptoms of Bipolar from those with ADHD. In contrast, ADD is never confused with Bipolar. Both ADHD and Bipolar children present irritability, hyperactivity, and distractibility, making the picture confusing. Bipolar children have serious symptoms, however, that are notably absent in ADHD; namely labile moods that alternate between excessively happy and highly irritable, grandiose behaviors, flight of ideas, intense temper rages, depression, and decreased need for sleep. Several studies have reported that over 80 percent of children who have childhood Bipolar Disorder also meet full criteria for ADHD. Researchers are studying whether ADHD may be a precursor to later development of Bipolar Disorder or if they coexist, or if ADHD symptoms are the first signs on the continuum of Bipolar Disorder. Studies are also finding a high incidence of ODD in children with Bipolar Disorder.

The first line of treatment for Bipolar Disorder is mood-stabilizing medication. Psychotherapy is an important adjunct treatment to help the child and family learn to cope with the ongoing symptoms and the damaging effects they have on the child's academic, social, and family life.

What is Developmental Coordination Disorder?

Developmental Coordination Disorder (DCD) is a childhood disorder characterized by poor coordination and clumsiness. Children with DCD have marked difficulties with gross and/or fine motor movement that interfere with their academic performance and/or daily life activities. Roughly 6 percent of school-age children have some degree of Developmental Coordination Disorder. Children with DCD may trip over their own feet, run into other children, have trouble holding objects, and have an unsteady gait, similar to the clumsiness seen in children with AD/HD.

Developmental Coordination Disorder may appear in conjunction with other learning disorders or may occur alone. Communication Disorders and Disorder of Written Expression are two of the learning disorders often associated with this condition. Children with ADHD are often poorly coordinated, some severe enough to be diagnosed with DCD.

Children with DCD are identified by parents and teachers as clumsy, awkward, and poor in athletics. Fine motor skills such as buttoning clothing and writing can be a challenge for these children. Gross motor skills such as running, hopping, kicking a ball, riding a bike, skating, and catching a ball may be noticeably delayed. Children are diagnosed with DCD if they fall below expectations for their age in these types of skills.

DCD is diagnosed and treated by occupational therapists, often provided by the public school special education services.

What should parents know about Developmental Coordination Disorder?

Children with Developmental Coordination Disorder can suffer related emotional problems due to their physical limitations. They avoid difficult tasks and activities with procrastination, refusal, or tantrums. These reactions are similar to the behaviors of children with AD/HD, so DCD may therefore not be diagnosed, as their behavior problems overshadow their motor problems.

Writing can be one of the most frustrating challenges. Children with fine motor problems write extremely large, write very messy, cannot write on a line, and have many erasures to the point of tearing the paper. Their frustration can result in avoiding school and homework, crying, and arguments about having to write—the very behaviors exhibited by children with AD/HD.

Gross motor movement problems tend to interfere with self-esteem and social relationships more than academic abilities. Children who are clumsy and uncoordinated are easily observed on the playground by their peers who reject them when it comes time to pick teammates for games. Embarrassment, frustration, and anger can result in these children engaging in many of the same inappropriate behaviors seen in children with AD/HD, including starting arguments, grabbing the ball in order to get attention, physical fights, and social isolation as they try to escape peer rejection and ridicule.

What are Enuresis and Encopresis?

Enuresis is a disorder of wetting the bed or clothing. It is not unusual for children with AD/HD to have enuresis. Primary enuresis is found in children who have never been dry for longer than six months. Secondary enuresis occurs in children who have achieved dryness for at least six months, and then begin to wet themselves. Nocturnal enuresis is more commonly known as bed-wetting, while diurnal enuresis occurs during the waking hours. Encopresis involves bowel movements outside the toilet in children aged four years or older.

Children and teens understandably do not like to admit to toileting problems and therefore we do not know the number of children and teens with enuresis and encopresis. Studies estimate that at age five, enuresis affects 5 to 10 percent of all children, with the majority being boys. The incidence drops significantly with age. By age ten, it affects 3 percent of boys and 2 percent of girls. About 1 percent of adolescents still experience enuresis. Encopresis is present in only 1 percent of five-year-olds and, as with enuresis, is more common in boys. Enuresis has very strong family ties, with 75 percent of those affected having a first-degree biological relative who also had the disorder.

Having enuresis or encopresis is associated with a higher incidence of coexisting behavioral symptoms.

What should parents know about Enuresis and Encopresis?

Rates of enuresis are significantly higher in boys with AD/HD, although researchers do not know why this is the case. Estimates for daytime enuresis are three times higher for boys with AD/HD and five times higher for nighttime enuresis than for non-disordered boys. It is not unusual for boys with AD/HD to wet the bed until ten or twelve years old.

Children eventually outgrow enuresis and encopresis, even without treatment. However, years of frustration between parent and child can have a very negative effect on the relationship and the child's self-esteem. Many children who wet the bed avoid sleepovers and overnight camps due to fear of being discovered by their peers as a bed wetter—which typically results in devastating ridicule and humiliation that is difficult to overcome—even after the problem no longer exists.

The emotional consequences of enuresis and encopresis make treatment necessary. However, no psychotherapy should be started until medical clearance is obtained by a pediatric urologist and/or gastroenterologist who can ensure there are no physical causes to the wetting or soiling.

If physical causes are ruled out, emotional causes need to be considered. Anxiety, changes in the family, and emotional trauma are commonly seen in children with secondary enuresis and encopresis.

Chapter 4

SUCCEEDING
IN SCHOOL

- Do children with AD/HD qualify for special education?
- What is Section 504?
- Who qualifies for Section 504?
- What is a Section 504 meeting?
- What are reasonable accommodations under Section 504?
- What should I do if my child is denied Section 504?
- What is the IDEA law for special education?
- Who qualifies for special education under IDEA?
- What qualifies a child with AD/HD as Other Health Impaired?
- What steps are necessary to obtain special education under IDEA?
- What tests are included in the evaluation for special education?
- What is an IEP?
- What should be included in the written IEP?
- What special education services are available?
- What if my child is denied special education services under IDEA?
- Can children with AD/HD be denied special education?
- Will the school accept an independent assessment?
- What are parents' responsibilities in the special education process?
- How can a special education advocate help?
- What if my child's school does not have special education?
- What if my child goes to a private school?
- Will special education stigmatize my child?
- What should I know about my child's special education records?
- Who can access my child's records?
- What are the exceptions to privacy of my child's records?
- Should I tell my child's teacher about his or her AD/HD?
- How can I find out how my child is doing in the classroom?
- Should my child repeat a grade to give him time to mature?
- How are behavior problems handled through special education?
- How are suspensions and expulsions handled for special education students?

Do children with AD/HD qualify for special education?

It was not until 1991 that children with AD/HD were considered disabled under federal law. Before the U.S. Department of Education formally included AD/HD under the umbrella of disability, children with AD/HD were *not* eligible for special education services.

Two federal laws, Section 504 and IDEA, now guarantee children with AD/HD a "free appropriate public education" in the "least restrictive environment." Free means the education must be of no cost to the parents and appropriate means that it must meet the individual needs of each child. The least restrictive environment means that children with disabilities are not to be segregated from their nondisabled peers simply because of their disability. If they are to be removed from their peers, it is only for the portion of their education that cannot be met in the "general" or "mainstream" classroom.

Each law has different procedures and criteria for eligibility and different services available. IDEA states that the child must have a disability that requires special education services. Section 504 has a lower threshold and requires only that the child need modifications and accommodations in order to take part in learning. All public schools across the nation that receive federal funds are required to follow these two federal laws.

What is Section 504?

Section 504 is the section of the Rehabilitation Act of 1973 that applies to persons with disabilities. It is a civil rights act that protects the civil rights of persons with disabilities, including AD/HD.

For practical purposes, what Section 504 means to you is that public schools cannot discriminate against your child and must make "reasonable accommodations and modifications" for your child's disability. It is designed to level the playing field for individuals with disabilities and to ensure that those with disabilities have the same access to learning that individuals without disabilities have.

For most students with AD/HD, the reason to obtain Section 504 is that the child does not need a special education setting, but is in need of accommodations and modifications in order to be successful in school. Section 504 makes allowances, modifications, and/or accommodations to help the child with AD/HD compensate in areas where her disorder causes a significant negative impact on her educational performance.

Children who have AD/HD but do not meet criteria under IDEA often are eligible for assistance under Section 504. If a child is qualified under IDEA he is automatically qualified under Section 504; however, the reverse is not true.

Who qualifies for Section 504?

A student is eligible for Section 504 if she meets the definition of a "qualified handicapped person." The student does not need to be eligible for special education under IDEA in order to be a "handicapped person" or to be protected and provided accommodations and modifications under Section 504. To qualify for Section 504, the child must:

- Be determined to have a physical or mental impairment that substantially limits one or more major life activities, including learning and behavior
- Have a record of having such an impairment or be regarded as having such impairment

In addition to a wide variety of physical disabilities and mental disorders, AD/HD is included in this legal definition. The term "major life activities" includes learning and, therefore, applies to the school setting.

Not every student with AD/HD will qualify for Section 504. Her AD/HD must be determined to substantially limit her learning. The school district is required, if requested by the parents, to determine if the child's AD/HD is substantially limiting her success in school. However, the evaluation is not required to be a full evaluation simply because a parent requests one. The school is allowed to determine that a prescreening meets the criteria for an evaluation.

What is a Section 504 meeting?

A Section 504 meeting is between parents and school personnel to discuss the child's eligibility for accommodations and modifications. The school may initiate the meeting after identifying the child as having a potential disability that is interfering with learning. However, more often than not, the parents identify the difficulties their child is having due to a disability.

Parents can request a Section 504 meeting to determine eligibility for accommodations and modifications by writing to the school principal. Once the meeting is scheduled, parents are invited to attend and take part along with the child's teachers and any school personnel familiar with the child.

Be prepared to present your case for why your child needs accommodations and modifications. Bring a list of your child's behaviors and how they impair his learning. While you are not obligated to come up with solutions, having a list of suggestions will be very helpful and will increase your child's chances of obtaining the highest number of necessary accommodations and modifications.

If your child is determined to be eligible under Section 504, the regulations require that there be a written plan that describes what those accommodations and modifications will be.

What are reasonable accommodations under Section 504?

As recipients of federal funding, under Section 504 public schools must make *reasonable* accommodations and modifications for the eligible child unless it can demonstrate that to do so would impose an undue hardship on the operation of its program. Accommodations and modifications should be designed to place the student who has a disability at an equal starting level with the nonhandicapped student.

For AD/HD children, Section 504 has been a saving grace, allowing the child to remain in the general education classroom, but be accommodated to ease his struggles. Some examples of accommodations and modifications for the AD/HD child in the main categories of impairment include:

- Attention:
    Move seat to front of class
    Allow extra time to complete projects
- Impulsiveness:
    Ignore calling out without raising hand
    Provide immediate praise or rewards
- Motor Activity:
    Provide short breaks between assignments
    Allow standing while working
- Organization and Planning:
    Keep second set of textbooks at home
    Provide assignment book

- Compliance:
    Post rules in classroom
    Maintain behavior modification system in the classroom
- Mood:
    Compliment positive behavior
    Focus on student's talents
- Socialization:
    Prompt appropriate social behavior
    Supervise closely during transitions
- Academic Skills:
    Allow extra time to complete tests
    Decrease amount of homework

What should I do if my child is denied Section 504?

Perhaps one of the most frustrating aspects of advocating for your child's education is to see each day how he struggles in school, only to be informed that he does not meet criteria for eligibility.

Impairment, in and of itself, does not qualify your child for protection under Section 504. The impairment must substantially limit one or more major life activities in order to qualify for Section 504. Under Section 504, your child must not only have at least one disorder, but that disorder must negatively influence his ability to learn and/or perform academically.

If you believe your child meets criteria for Section 504 and he has been denied accommodations and modifications, you have a right to appeal this decision to the school. Each school district has its own appeal process. You can begin the appeal process by asking your child's school for a printed copy of the district's policies and procedures for Section 504. This written document may be titled "policies," "procedures," "safeguards," "parental rights," or a similar name. The appeal process should be outlined in the written document and it should be relatively easy for you to appeal the denial.

What is the IDEA law for special education?

IDEA is the federal law that governs special education services. IDEA stands for Individuals with Disabilities Education Act. This law protects students who need special education due to a disability. The law states that a child is entitled to a Free and Appropriate Education (FAPE) in the "least restrictive environment." To the greatest extent possible, the child protected by IDEA is to be educated in the mainstream classroom. IDEA thus prevents children with disabilities from being unnecessarily segregated from their nondisabled peers.

Under IDEA, children who are identified as having a potential disability are entitled to an evaluation at the school district's expense. Either a teacher or parent may identify the child as having a potential disability. Parents knowing or suspecting their child has AD/HD is not sufficient to require the school to perform an evaluation; the disorder must have an adverse effect on "educational performance." Educational performance refers to much more than your child's grades. It encompasses your child's complete functioning in all aspects of school, including his ability to behave, get along with peers, and complete work, among many other abilities.

The most recent version of the law, Individuals with Disabilities Education Improvement Act of 2004 (IDEA 2004) went into effect in July 2005. Changes were made with the goal of improving the quality of education for students with disabilities. Interpreting the changes in IDEA 2004 is best done by a special education advocate or attorney, especially for those students who have yet to have an IEP. In many cases the changes will have little or no affect on children who have an existing IEP.

Who qualifies for special education under IDEA?

Children between the ages of three and twenty-one years, who have one or more of the eligible specific disabilities and who require special education because of that disability can qualify for services under IDEA. Simply having a disability does not make someone eligible for services. The child must have a need for services because of the disability. Many children with AD/HD, despite the disorder, do not have their educational performance or school behavior affected by their disorder. Such children would not be eligible for special education services under IDEA.

The eligible disabilities are limited to:

- Autism
- Hearing impairments including deafness
- Mental retardation
- Multiple disabilities
- Orthopedic impairments
- Emotional disturbance
- Specific learning disability
- Speech or language impairments
- Traumatic brain injury
- Visual impairments including blindness
- Other health impairment (includes AD/HD)

Children with AD/HD who qualify under IDEA are likely to have a history of significant problems with completing class work, following rules, disrupting the class, conflicts with peers, and returning homework, among others.

What qualifies a child with AD/HD as Other Health Impaired?

For years, schools denied special education for AD/HD children, justifying their exclusion due to an absence of a learning disorder. Federal education laws now require AD/HD to be recognized by schools as a disability.

Children with AD/HD who qualify for special education under IDEA will be classified as "Other Health Impaired" (OHI). However, having a diagnosis of AD/HD alone is not sufficient and unless there is a specific need, a child with AD/HD can be disqualified for special education under IDEA.

The following are the specific criteria necessary to meet eligibility as OHI.

- The child must have a diagnosis of AD/HD and the disorder must have led to limited alertness in academic tasks.
- The effects of AD/HD must be chronic or acute.
- The effects of AD/HD must have an adverse effect on educational performance, including grades, achievement test scores, behavior problems, impaired or inappropriate social relations, or impaired work skills.
- The student requires special education services to address the AD/HD and its effects.

What steps are necessary to obtain special education under IDEA?

If you believe your child is in need of special education services, send a written request for an evaluation to the school principal. Each state sets its own period in which the school must respond to your request. For example, in California the school has fifteen calendar days to respond. Once parental consent is given for the assessment, the school then has fifty calendar days to complete it. Parents should check their state department of education website to determine the period in which their school must respond and evaluate.

Your child's school will either deny your request to assess or invite you to attend an "assessment" or "student study team" meeting. The meeting takes place to discuss the rationale and need for an assessment. If an assessment is granted, you will receive a written assessment plan, which you are to review and sign to consent for the assessment to take place. Some schools will skip the meeting and directly send you a written assessment plan.

An assessment will likely include:

- Individually administered standardized academic achievement test
- Teacher observations
- Review of classroom performance
- Speech and language assessment
- Social-emotional assessment
- Cognitive ability/intelligence assessment

What tests are included in the evaluation for special education?

Typically, the school psychologist will select a battery of tests to measure various areas of a child's functioning. Additional specialists will administer tests that are outside the realm of academics and behavior. A speech pathologist will use speech and language tests. A nurse will screen for vision and hearing deficits. If appropriate, an occupational therapist will assess fine and gross motor functioning.

Behavioral functioning is assessed by standardized questionnaires completed by parents and the teacher. Academic achievement is assessed by a standardized test administered face to face to measure the grade level achieved by your child in a wide variety of academic skills.

In order to test for a specific learning disorder, a child's intellectual/cognitive ability must be measured. Some schools achieve this by administering an IQ test. However, years ago, a court ruling found that IQ tests discriminated against African American children, causing most schools to abandon IQ tests. While nothing legally prohibits schools from using IQ tests to determine intelligence, most schools opt to use alternative tests to estimate cognitive ability.

School psychologists do not use test data to make a diagnosis of any disorder or disability. Results are used solely to determine eligibility, placement, and goals.

What is an IEP?

Once your child has been assessed by the school, you will be invited to attend the IEP meeting. IEP stands for Individualized Education Plan. In this meeting, you will meet with school personnel to discuss the assessment results and determine if your child is eligible for special education under IDEA. The invitation to the IEP must be given at least ten days in advance and scheduled at a mutually convenient time for the parents and school personnel. Parents have a right to reschedule the IEP if necessary.

The IEP meeting must include:

- Parents
- A teacher who is familiar with the student
- A special education teacher
- A school professional who is qualified to explain the test data
- A school representative who is able to authorize special education

If your child is eligible for special education, an IEP will be written. The school is obligated to provide only what is documented in the IEP. Do not accept a verbal promise of anything related to your child's education. You may take the IEP home with you to review. Carefully read the IEP and sign it only when you agree it is appropriate for your child's education. If you do not agree to a small part of the IEP, you may ask your school if they have an "informal dispute resolution," where minor disagreements can be quickly settled. If your school does not have such a process or if you are in disagreement with the IEP as a whole, your next step is to file for "due process," a formal process where you will either have mediation or a hearing in order to resolve the disagreement.

What should be included in the written IEP?

In addition to the IEP meeting, an IEP is also a written document that describes the educational, developmental, and behavioral support the child with a disability will receive. The school must supply what is written in the IEP. Contrarily, if it is not written in the IEP, the school does not have to provide it. An IEP must include:

- The child's specific eligibility for special education
- The child's present level of educational performance and how the child's disability affects their involvement and progress in the general curriculum
- Measurable goals to meet the child's needs, enabling the child to be involved in and progress with the general curriculum
- A statement of the special education and related services and supplemental aids and services
- Placement, with a description of the educational placement as the least restrictive environment
- Program accommodations and modifications or supports for the school personnel that will be provided for the child to advance appropriately towards attaining the annual goals
- An explanation of the extent to which the child will not participate with nondisabled children in the regular class

The IEP is reviewed annually to reestablish eligibility, evaluate progress, and make any necessary modifications.

What special education services are available?

Special education is to be provided in the least restrictive environment. This means that your child should be educated in the general education classroom to the furthest extent possible. The range of special education placements includes "full inclusion" in the regular classroom, "resource specialist program" where your child may go to a specialized classroom for a particular subject, and "special day class" where the child is educated full time with other disabled students.

In addition to placement, there is also a variety of related services (sometimes called Designated Instructional Services or DIS) available under IDEA. Your child will be provided only the related services deemed necessary for a FAPE. Some of the available services include:

- Assistive technology
- Speech therapy
- Occupational therapy
- Educational therapy
- Counseling
- Medical services
- Parent counseling and training
- Physical therapy
- Transportation
- Psychological services

In a few very severe cases where a child cannot receive a FAPE, he may qualify for a nonpublic school. These schools provide specialized services for children with specific disabilities. In the most extreme cases where a child is not safe in the home due to her disability and therefore cannot receive a FAPE while remaining home, residential placement may be available.

What if my child is denied special education under IDEA?

Children can be denied special education under IDEA at various points in the process. Your request for an evaluation may be denied. Your child may be evaluated but found ineligible. Or, you may not agree with the goals, objectives, services, or placement the school offers.

Parents may appeal a denial. However, a denial is unlikely to be overturned without evidence that your child's AD/HD has an adverse effect on his educational performance, including grades, achievement test scores, behavior problems, impaired or inappropriate social relations, or impaired work skills.

The first step in appealing the school's denial is to informally request a meeting with an official from the school district to discuss your child's eligibility. If this is not successful, the next step is to file for a "due process hearing."

A due process hearing is a formal legal process that varies from state to state. Details on how to file and what steps to take are spelled out in a document provided by each school district, usually entitled "procedurals safeguards." The hearing procedure will involve the filing of motions, presentation of evidence, and possible testimony. You should not attempt to file for a due process hearing without an attorney.

Can children with AD/HD be denied special education?

It is quite common for schools to deny special education services for children with AD/HD. Many children do not even get approved for an evaluation. Schools justify their denial of services by citing the fact that the child is of average or above IQ and has no apparent learning disorder based upon her standardized academic achievement scores. Since most children with AD/HD are average or above IQ and only about 10 percent have a diagnosable learning disorder, the majority of parents raising AD/HD children will face this frustrating battle.

Parents of AD/HD children know that their child is struggling in school, no matter how intelligent their child is. The child passing her classes is often more a reflection of her parents' persistence and dedication than the child's effort, knowledge, and performance. Schools often fail to recognize the invisible, immeasurable disorder of AD/HD, regard it as laziness, and do not view it as a disability that requires special assistance.

The best way to combat this unjustified denial of services is to know the criteria for services under IDEA and Section 504. If your child meets criteria, then she is eligible and the school must obey the law and provide services.

Will the school accept an independent assessment?

While schools are required to consider outside sources of information about your child, they are not mandated to agree with it. Even if you have a private evaluation, your child's school will conduct their own evaluation.

There are benefits to seeking an independent assessment. It can be done quickly, in comparison to the school district's waiting period. They are also likely to be more thorough than the assessment done by the school. An IQ test can be administered, which provides far more information than the general cognitive assessment the school will use. You will also be provided with a detailed written report of the test scores and findings that your evaluator will explain to you in a face-to-face meeting. The only downside to a private evaluation is the cost that you may bear, which can range from $1,000 to $3,000.

Your private evaluator may reach a more complete or different understanding of your child's disability than found by the school personnel. However, if your child is determined to be eligible for special education, it is not so important that they agree with your evaluator. On the other hand, if your private evaluation indicates that your child qualifies for special education but the school denies eligibility, you may appeal the denial.

What are parents' responsibilities in the special education process?

As a parent, you must play an active role in your child's education. With increasing numbers of children undergoing evaluation for special education, it is more important than ever that parents become informed about the evaluation process, services available, and their rights. Gone are the days for parents to simply turn their child's education over to the school. Some schools are excellent sources of information about special education, while others are sorely lacking. It is up to parents to stay informed and advocate for their child's needs.

Being active in your child's education includes keeping thorough records. Make a file for each year of your child's education. Place report cards, annual academic achievement test scores, notes from teachers, IEPs, Section 504 accommodation plans, and any additional records regarding your child's education in this file. Document all phone calls you have with any school personnel. Organized and complete records will be invaluable in your annual IEP and Section 504 accommodation meeting.

You are also responsible for keeping in frequent communication with your child's teacher. Going to the teacher with a teamwork approach will be well received. A "how can I help you help my child?" approach usually sets the stage for a cooperative relationship.

How can a special education advocate help?

The special education process is unknown territory for most parents. Parents are at a disadvantage in the school meetings where the policies, procedures, laws, and language of special education are known to every committee member except them. While some schools are very helpful with the special education procedures, others withhold information, leaving parents feeling lost.

For every parent who is able to obtain special education for her child on her own, another was unsuccessful. Too many parents decide they can "go it alone" and figure they will spend the money for an advocate if things do not turn out their way. This can be penny-wise and pound-foolish. Saving the money by not hiring an advocate costs your child another year of not getting her educational needs met.

Parents can best obtain special education by seeking consult with a special education advocate before the 504 or IEP meeting. These specialists know the special education laws. They know the school district personnel, what services are available, how to interpret the assessment results, and can advise you regarding your child's needs. They accompany you to the school meetings, speak on your behalf, and are very successful at getting your child the services he needs.

What if my child's school does not have special education?

Federal law requires that children who qualify for special education be provided access to the necessary placements and services. A school cannot escape their legal obligation to provide a free appropriate public education to every child by simply saying they do not have special education services.

Most school districts are prepared for situations when a child's special needs cannot be met by the school. For large school districts in highly populated cities, the provision of services and placement is usually not a problem. If your child's school does not have the appropriate classroom placement or services, the correct setting likely exists in a nearby school, to which your child will be provided transportation. If your child has needs for special services that are not ordinarily provided by her school, the district may bring in a specialist to your child's campus. In smaller areas, two or three school districts will often work together to share resources.

If your child's school district refuses to provide necessary placement or services by claiming they do not have what your child needs, they are in violation of the law. Parents in this situation are best advised to consult with an advocate or lawyer.

What if my child goes to a private school?

Children with disabilities who are in a private school by parental choice still have rights and access to special education under IDEA. Procedures for evaluation and services are the same as for children enrolled in the local public school. The privately schooled child is entitled to a "services plan" that describes the specific special education and related services the school district will provide. The services plan is similar to an IEP. A representative from the private school must provide input or attend the services plan meeting; however, they do not have to provide any special education services.

Services provided to the disabled child may be at the private school, but are not required to take place there. If services are provided off-site from the private school, the school district must supply necessary transportation. Transportation is only required from the private school to the location of the special education service, not from home to the private school.

Even though services are available for AD/HD children in private school, it is usually not the best solution. These children typically function better in a nonpublic school designed solely for AD/HD children or in a public school with services for the AD/HD child.

Will special education stigmatize my child?

When parents think of special education, they usually reflect back to unpleasant childhood memories of special education students at their school. Children with disabilities were kept completely isolated from the general education students and were not allowed to share recess and lunch periods, participate in general PE classes, and were prevented from attending school social activities.

Fortunately, special education has come a long way since today's parents were in school. Children are included in the general education setting to the greatest extent possible and are no longer segregated. Still, parents worry about their child's self-esteem if they are "labeled" as a special needs child. This worry usually lives more in the imagination of the parents than in the self-image of the child. When parents come to understand that labeling a child as a special education student is a necessary entry procedure to obtaining services, they are able to decrease their fears.

General education and special education teachers are aware of the teasing that special education students may receive from their nondisabled peers and typically work to teach all students that special education is not negative, and is just a different way for students to learn. Parents can reinforce this with their emotional support of their child.

What should I know about my child's special education records?

Schools are required by federal and state laws to maintain certain records and to have them available to you upon request. The federal law Family Educational Rights and Privacy Act (FERPA) establishes minimum requirements for maintaining, protecting, and providing access to school records. State laws may have additional protections.

Under FERPA, parents have a right to all files and documents maintained by the school system that contain information related to their child. This includes any documents that identify your child by name, social security number, school identification number, or other data that make the records traceable back to your child.

Your child's records will be broken into several files. The cumulative file includes personal identification, academic achievement test scores, teacher reports, and report cards. The confidential file holds written reports from the school's evaluations, any evaluation reports and records you provided, IEPs, written documents between yourself and school personnel, and reports from IEP team members.

Some schools will keep a compliance file that holds documents that demonstrate the school's compliance with IDEA. This would include reports of eligibility meetings and correspondence between the school and parents. Finally, some schools keep a discipline file where they hold records regarding suspensions and expulsion.

Who can access my child's records?

Special education records are quite secure and there is little need to worry about negative consequences from having a special education file.

All documents related to special education are permanently kept in a file separate from your child's usual academic records. These files are marked "confidential" and are accessible only by school personnel who have a "need to know." Special education teachers, school counselors, and any specialist providing special education services to your child are considered as having a need to know. Teachers who will not be addressing your child's special education needs have no cause to read your child's confidential file.

Only parents or guardians have the legal authority to allow the release of their child's school records, including the confidential file. Once the child turns eighteen, the authority transfers to her. When the parents or adult child request the school records to be released, only the general education file is sent. Only with specific written request can the confidential file be released.

Parents and the senior high school student will want to consider releasing the most recent IEP to the student's college of choice. Colleges provide 504 accommodations that may assist your child in her college education.

What are the exceptions to the privacy of my child's records?

The federal laws of FERPA and IDEA protect your child's records from being shown to anyone without your written consent. However, as with all records, there are always exceptions. The law allows for access to your child's school record by the following individuals or agencies:

- School officials with a legitimate educational interest
- School officials in the district to which your child intends to transfer
- Certain state and national education agencies for purposes of enforcing federal laws
- Anyone to whom a state statute requires the school to report information to
- Accrediting and research organizations helping the school, provided they guarantee confidentiality
- Student financial aid officials
- People who have court orders, provided the school makes reasonable efforts to notify the parents prior to releasing the records
- Law enforcement and judicial authorities in certain cases

What most parents are concerned about are potential colleges and employers gaining access to the confidential file. Unless specifically authorized in writing to do so, the school district may not release the confidential file to a college or employer.

Should I tell my child's teacher about his or her AD/HD?

At the beginning of the new school year, parents and children are optimistic that the child will have a fresh start. Parents wonder if they should tell the new teacher that their child has AD/HD; questioning if knowing the child has a disorder will bias the teacher against their child. They hold out hope that the fresh start will last and if the teacher is not aware of the disorder, the child's problems will not be discovered.

Unfortunately, this rarely happens. Children cannot hide their AD/HD. The symptoms are certain to show after the initial honeymoon phase of the new school year is over. Not telling the teacher leaves her to guess what is causing the child's difficulties.

Rather than blindsiding the teacher, you can be far more helpful to her and to your child by informing her right up front. A note to the teacher indicating that your child has AD/HD and a request to meet with her in the first few weeks of school is suggested. Prepare information for the meeting, providing the teacher with a list of behaviors she is likely to observe in your child and a list of proposed solutions that you and prior teachers have found helpful.

How can I find out how my child is doing in the classroom?

In the absence of a note sent home from the teacher, parents assume things are going well. Come report card time, parents are often unpleasantly surprised.

While some teachers will make frequent contact through notes or phone calls to parents, unfortunately the majority are simply too busy to do so. Unless teachers are asked to report progress, many wait until report card time, far too long to inform parents about their AD/HD child.

If your child has a written IEP or a Section 504 accommodation plan, request that the method and frequency of contact between yourself and the teacher be written into the plan. The teacher must comply with what is written in either plan, regardless of how busy he is.

Rather than wait for the teacher to make contact, parents of AD/HD children should contact the teacher early in the school year and ask what method he would prefer to keep you informed about your child's school work and behavior. Have a plan in mind that would be easy for the teacher to use. Email, voice mail, or a behavior chart can be quick methods that will not burden the teacher's time.

Should my child repeat a grade to give him time to mature?

Children with AD/HD are often emotionally and socially delayed at a minimum of one to two years. Behaviors their peers have outgrown persist in AD/HD children well beyond what is expected. This immaturity may lead parents to consider having their child repeat a grade in order to give him time to "catch up" to his classmates. This may sound good in theory, but in reality, it does not work and is not supported by research.

Holding a child back for a year might work if he were evenly delayed one year in all areas. However, AD/HD children have very scattered emotional development. A child may have the vocabulary of an adult, the frustration tolerance of a three-year-old, and the social skills of a second-grade student. Given the large gaps in emotional maturity, there is no one grade level that will even the playing field for the AD/HD child.

Children do not "catch up" or outgrow the symptoms throughout their childhood much less in one school year. Holding an AD/HD child back one year fails to bring about emotional growth. The best solution is to seek an IEP or Section 504 accommodation plan.

How are behavior problems handled through special education?

Teachers generally try to motivate children to perform well and cooperate with classroom rules with the use of praise, encouragement, and privileges. For many children with AD/HD, these behavioral techniques are insufficient and the child is often found to disrupt the teacher and classmates. For such children, either the parent or teacher may request the assistance of a behaviorist to perform a "behavioral functional assessment."

In this special type of assessment, a behaviorist will observe your child in the classroom, looking for when the problem behavior arises, what triggers it, what consequences are used, and how effective the consequences are. The behaviorist is looking for underlying causes of the problem behavior to determine if it can be prevented.

If the behaviorist determines that a behavior modification program is likely to be successful in decreasing or eliminating the behavior, she will design a plan. The goal is to modify the behavior so that the child will be able to remain in the general education classroom. The behaviorist will train the teacher in how to implement the plan. The plan will generally involve one or more specific behaviors with methods to prevent them, rewards to give, and methods to keep track of success.

How are suspensions and expulsions handled for special education students?

Children with ADHD are more likely to get suspended or expelled from school than their ADD and nondisabled peers. Under IDEA, there are specific rules regarding suspensions and expulsions for special education students that protect them from excessive and unproductive disciplinary action. Each state sets a maximum number of days a special education student may be suspended. California law, for example, sets a maximum of ten days.

Special education students may not be expelled from a school district if their misbehavior is due to their disability or if they were inappropriately placed in their academic setting. A "manifestation hearing" is held when a school district wants to expel a student. The hearing determines if the child's behavior that caused the suspension was due to the disability, if the IEP and special education services the child has are appropriate in relation to the offending behavior, whether or not the child understands the effects and consequences of his behavior, and whether or not the child is able to control the problem behavior. The hearing is a formal legal process and parents are therefore advised to seek the services of a special education attorney to assist them.

If the disability is determined to be a factor in the problem behavior, or if the IEP is determined to be inadequate to address the problem behavior, then the child cannot be held to the same standards and arbitrarily suspended or switched to another program. Instead, the school must change its approach to the problem behavior in order to prevent it from happening again.

If parents disagree with the manifestation determination, they may request a due process hearing. Until such time, the child has a "stay put" order and is allowed to remain in his current placement until proceedings are concluded. Exceptions to this stay put order include a child bringing a weapon or drugs to school, or presents as a danger to himself or others.

Under Section 504, the child is not given the same protection. The school does not have to keep the child in school while they perform an assessment for the offending behavior.

Under the 1997 IDEA, the district has the burden to prove that the behavior that is causing the expulsion is not a "manifestation of" the child's disability. Under the 2004 IDEA, the burden is expected to switch to the parents who will have to prove that the behavior was a manifestation of their child's disability.

Chapter 5

HOMEWORK

- Why is homework so difficult for AD/HD children?
- What is the purpose of homework?
- Does homework improve learning?
- Are teachers giving increasing amounts of homework?
- Why is there so much emphasis on homework?
- How much homework is reasonable?
- What if my child's teacher is giving excessive homework?
- Do activities outside of school affect children's success on homework?
- What is my role in homework?
- What structure will best help my child with homework?
- What if activities prevent homework from being structured?
- How can I make homework more exciting?
- How can a homework club help?
- Can a tutor help?
- What if I am unable to afford a tutor?
- How do I get my child organized?
- How do I get my child to plan ahead for projects?
- How can I find out what my child's homework is?
- How can I get my child to use an assignment book?
- Should I give my child breaks during homework?
- Are there any devices that can aid my child in homework?
- Where should my child do homework?
- Are there strategies to decrease my child's homework anxiety?
- Should I punish my child for not doing homework?
- When should my child be able to do his own homework?
- How can teachers help with homework?
- What if nothing seems to help?
- How can Section 504 accommodations and modifications help with homework?

Why is homework so difficult for AD/HD children?

For most parents with an AD/HD child, homework is the bane of their existence. For children without AD/HD, homework is no picnic either, but they do not spend hours battling with their parents over it. The entire process of homework from the time it is assigned until the time it is turned in is complex and involves behaviors that are challenging for AD/HD children.

To start, the child must hear the assignment, understand it, and write it down correctly. She must decide what items she needs to bring home and put them in her backpack, remembering to take it home. Resisting the temptation to lie about having homework, she must resign herself to do it, knowing she will miss out on fun. She has to unpack the backpack, review her assignment book, prioritize assignments, and organize the materials.

Next comes actually doing the work. She must pay attention, focus, and resist distractions. She needs to exert effort on boring and tedious tasks and make herself slow down so her work is legible. Once done, she has to pack her backpack, being sure her homework makes it in. Her final step is to turn the homework in.

Each step presents a challenge and opportunity for problems and conflict.

What is the purpose of homework?

The answer to this question seems obvious: homework helps children learn. However, this simple answer is incomplete and not exactly accurate.

Homework should serve different purposes, depending on your child's grade level and individual abilities. For primary grades, homework is largely used to improve reading and to review skills taught in class. Intermediate grade students are given homework to continue with reading skills and to improve a child's ability to remember, understand, and practice skills learned in class. Homework for middle school students provides practice of skills taught in class, an opportunity to learn new information, and to demonstrate knowledge obtained. High school students have the added goal of using homework as a way to apply learned principles to new situations, as well as engage in independent learning at home.

Homework is also designed to teach, reinforce, and enhance lifelong skills of responsibility, independent learning, time management, organization, planning, perseverance, and self-discipline.

Homework also provides parents with an understanding of what their child is learning in class. Teachers expect parents of kindergarten through second grade students to be actively involved in their child's homework. Instilling a love of learning is a primary goal of homework for early elementary students.

Does homework improve learning?

It would be logical to assume that one of the major purposes of homework is to increase your child's learning. After all, if she is not learning by doing homework, what is the purpose?

That is exactly what researchers have asked. In a review of over 120 studies on the effectiveness of homework, researchers found that learning, as measured on academic achievement tests, was increased by doing assigned homework for higher grade levels. High school students doing homework outperformed their peers who were not assigned homework 75 percent of the time. In middle school, this positive effect dropped close to 35 percent. Most interesting, however, was the consistent finding across studies that in elementary school, there was very little difference in the academic achievement of students who did homework compared to those who were not assigned homework. When researchers examined whether or not the length of time doing homework has an impact on academic achievement test scores, the findings followed the same pattern of only the higher grade students benefiting from spending more time on homework.

These findings certainly raise the question about the usefulness of homework for elementary students. Are all those hours of conflict with your child over homework worth it?

Are teachers giving increasing amounts of homework?

If you think that your child is assigned far more homework than you were in childhood, you are not alone. Parents are as overwhelmed with homework as their child is. However, researchers say that children being made to do hours of homework each day is a myth.

According to 2003 "The Brown Center Report on American Education 2003," there have been increases in the past two decades, but they are modest and relatively insignificant. Surveys show that students at all grade levels across the nation are now spending twenty-three minutes more on homework each week than they did in 1981. In 1981, students spent an average of one hour and fifty-three minutes on homework each week. In 1997, the time spent on homework increased to two hours and sixteen minutes. With an average of four nights of homework per week, this translates into about six additional minutes per night; hardly a dramatic increase.

Significant increases, however, were found in first through third grade students. The average primary grade student has gone from a nightly average of thirteen minutes of homework to thirty-two minutes.

Even though everyone else's child is not spending hours on homework each night, chances are your AD/HD child is.

Why is there so much emphasis on homework?

Despite national research findings that today's children are no more burdened with homework than their parents were, many parents would beg to differ. It is not unusual for parents to report their kindergartner has one hour of homework each night or that their third grader is up until 10:00 p.m. completing his assignments.

Our success-driven society has adopted the belief that education is the only way to success. Pressure to read before kindergarten has parents frantic that maybe they should have their child wait another year to start school so their child will have an advantage over the other kids.

Many parents see a lot of homework as a sign that their child is at a "good" school. Homework has erroneously been identified as the pathway to success, believing the more the better. Homework appears to the success-driven parent as the golden ticket to college, and unless their child goes to college, they are doomed for an adult life of minimum-wage jobs.

Teachers have also succumbed to societal pressure for more homework. Pressure to meet government standards on academic achievement tests has many teachers using homework as a method to teach what they do not have time for in class.

How much homework is reasonable?

The U.S. Department of Education and the National Parent Teacher Association recommend that the amount of homework assigned is equivalent to ten minutes per grade level.

First graders should have ten minutes; third graders, thirty minutes; and sixth grade students, sixty minutes. Increasing amounts of homework is advised for middle and high school students. Additional time for nightly reading is strongly recommended for primary grade students. Neither the U.S. Department of Education or the NPTA recommend homework for kindergarten children.

Ten minutes of homework each night per grade level is a reasonable expectation for most children with AD/HD. Even if your child does not complete all of his assigned homework, if he spends ten minutes per grade level, he is meeting the recommended time spent.

The majority of children with AD/HD can, however, be expected to take at least two to three times as long to complete the same amount of work as their classmates. As the child advances into fourth, fifth, and sixth grades, the length of time to complete the standard amount of homework becomes quite significant. The distress this causes can overshadow the benefits of homework. How much homework time is reasonable for your child is best decided with the help of your child's teacher.

What if my child's teacher is giving excessive homework?

The guidelines set out by the NPTA and U.S. Department of Education are recommendations only. Your child's school district and teacher will ultimately decide how much homework is assigned. Excessive is in the eye of the beholder. What one parent views as excessive, another may view as "just right" and another as "too little."

Excessive should be defined not by quantity but by your child's performance on homework. If your fourth grade son completes two hours each day with only minor struggles, then it is not excessive. If your first grader has daily tantrums and takes two hours to complete what other students finish in fifteen minutes, then, for him, the amount is excessive.

The first step to take if you think your child is detrimentally affected by her homework is to request a meeting with her teacher. Bring with you samples of your child's homework with notes on how long it took to complete and what it took to get it done. Follow suggestions the teacher offers and schedule a follow-up meeting.

If several suggestions fail to bring about a better response and performance to homework, then a written request for Section 504 accommodations and modifications is your next step.

Do activities outside of the school affect children's success on homework?

Television has long been accused of being the culprit of many of children's problems. While it indeed creates conflicts when children have to abandon a program to do homework, there have been inconsistent findings that television watching causes a decrease in academic success. Some studies show a decrease in grades and academic achievement test scores for those students who watch increased amounts of television on school nights. Other studies, however, show no such relationship.

Extracurricular activities concern parents about the time they take away from homework. With most AD/HD children having homework and extracurricular activities, it can be difficult for you to balance the amount of time your child spends with each. Studies have shown that children who participate in outside activities actually have increased academic achievement test scores and higher teacher assigned grades. This is particularly true of activities that are connected to the child's school. Similar results have been found for middle and high school students who have a part-time job. This positive relationship does reverse when there are so many outside activities that they interfere with completing homework, finishing projects, and regular school hours.

What is my role in homework?

How many times have you asked, "whose homework is it anyway?" Do you feel like you actually earned the grade on the science project? Have you spent too many late nights typing your child's book report while he slept? If you've wondered where to draw the line between help and actually doing your child's homework, you are not the only one. Parents of AD/HD children very often find themselves doing far more of their children's homework than other parents do.

A good guideline to follow is to keep your role focused on providing the structured time, setting, and materials needed to do homework while giving encouragement and motivation to stay on task. Surely you do not want your child to fail, but it is important to remember that homework is your child's work, not your work. The purpose of homework is not to "get it done," but to learn something. The grade for the assignment is your child's grade to earn, not your grade. The goal is the learning, not the earning.

What structure will best help my child with homework?

Structure and routine is the name of the game for homework for all children, but particularly for AD/HD students. Without a predictable approach to homework, conflict is guaranteed.

The ideal time for children to do homework is right after returning home from school. The time it takes to get from school to home, change clothes, use the restroom, and have a snack is sufficient to give your child a mental break from school. Allow a fixed time of no more than thirty minutes relaxation time between arriving home and starting homework.

Homework is to be done before anything else. Absolutely no privileges are earned until after you determine that homework has been done satisfactorily.

Since AD/HD children need direct supervision during homework time for years beyond their peers, choose a place in the home where you can be right next to or close to your child. The dining room table is a favorite location for many families.

A basket on the table that has all the supplies she could ever possibly need will prevent her from wasting time leaving the room to look for necessary items. Calm and quiet in the household will decrease opportunities for distraction.

What if activities prevent homework from being structured?

Your child's extracurricular activities are bound to disrupt the ideal structure of doing homework right after school. His schedule likely varies from day to day between therapy, sports, tutoring, and other activities. It is important that each day has a structure to it. It may not be the same structure every day, but your child should know what the routine for homework is each day of the week.

Working parents have the challenge of not being home to help with homework right after school. By the time they get home, it is usually dinnertime. Starting homework in the evening is, unfortunately, the worst time for parent and child. Both are tired from the day's work and more work is the last thing either want to do.

You can enlist the help of your after-school caretakers to assist you in providing a routine in your absence. The same structure of homework before play can work wherever your child spends his afternoons. Play and/or small rewards upon completing homework, as well as privileges once he gets home, can provide the necessary motivation your child needs to do his homework before you pick him up.

How can I make homework more exciting?

Knowing that AD/HD children are exceedingly easy to bore and exceptionally hard to motivate, be creative in the methods you employ. Once you find something that works, it may last only a short while and you will have to move on to something else to keep his attention and motivation.

Some solutions parents have found successful include changing the location of where homework is done. On sunny days, go to a neighborhood park and on cold days, the local library. The excitement of going to a college library can plant seeds of education as a desirable pursuit.

Drilling with flashcards can be done while you take a walk together. Reading can be done while taking a bubble bath. Studying for tests can be done in a mock interview on the family video camera and watched for fun. Practice spelling words with paint and a paintbrush. Double a cookie recipe to practice multiplication tables. Watch the movie version of an assigned book to stimulate thoughts for a book report and increase interest in history. Play a favorite board game, but replace game cards with flashcards. Reverse roles and have your child drill you on study materials.

How can a homework club help?

A homework club can be a formal club organized by your child's school or an informal club created by parents. Homework clubs provide a place for your child to do homework and receive assistance from an adult.

Parents can work with their child's school to create a homework club on campus. However, if your school has restrictions preventing them from doing so, parents can easily establish one outside of the school.

Chances are you are not the only parent that has problems getting your child to do homework. Many parents would be overjoyed at the thought of someone organizing a homework club. The more parents involved the better, but it really only takes two to get the job done.

If the school is not able to provide you with a room on campus, check with a nearby church, assembly hall, or community college. Your home can also provide the setting.

Parents volunteering in the homework club provide supervision while children complete their work. Keeping the children on task and giving them direction, help, and encouragement provides AD/HD children the support they need. Having treats, small rewards, and games to play after the work is done will provide the incentive for the children to do their work.

Can a tutor help?

A tutor can be a salvation for a parent trying to get their AD/HD child to do his homework. Even for AD/HD children who are highly intelligent and do not need extra help to learn concepts, a tutor can save the parent-child relationship. The majority of AD/HD children will not argue, throw a tantrum, and battle with a tutor like they will with you. That alone makes a tutor worth every penny.

Tutors generally have a wide range of experience, from teachers with a master's degree in special education, to college students, to smart high school students. The rates they charge can run from $7 an hour for a high school student to $50 an hour for a teacher. Not every AD/HD child needs a $50-an-hour special education teacher to help with his homework. Only those that have learning disabilities need the high level of expertise of a master's level person. Most children with AD/HD simply need someone to sit with them and keep them focused. A college student or college-bound high school student can easily do this.

Find a tutor who your child likes, looks forward to seeing, and wants to please. The bond your child has with the tutor will have a large impact on how successful the tutoring is. Let the tutor give the rewards for completion of homework to strengthen the bond.

What if I am unable to afford a tutor?

Ideally, it would be nice for your child to have a tutor every day. However, few parents can afford it on a regular basis. Creativity can make up where money leaves off and free tutoring can be found.

Find another parent who has a child struggling with homework and you can trade off tutoring with the other parent. You don't need any special skills other than the ability to sit calmly with the child and provide encouragement, redirection, and support. Planning a fun activity immediately afterward will encourage both children to complete their work.

Teens and college students excited about a future career helping children are often eager to obtain experience working with special needs students. Offer a letter of recommendation to a college or graduate school in exchange for tutoring. People innately have a need to volunteer to help others. Be creative and approach organizations where you might find a person willing to donate time to help your child. Women's clubs, retirement homes, local charity clubs, senior scouts, and religious institutions are places to start.

How do I get my child organized?

If your child is like most children with AD/HD, her backpack and bedroom look like long forgotten science experiments. Organization is not only an area of weakness for AD/HD children, it's also just not a priority.

Resign yourself to helping your child with organization for years longer than you would otherwise think appropriate. You will have to organize her school belongings far more frequently than you would otherwise think is necessary.

At homework time, you may have to help organize the materials and the order of the work to be done. You will have to assist in packing the backpack. Homework is less likely to get lost if you supply a plastic file folder with a Velcro closure that is marked and used solely for homework ready to be turned in.

Color coding is an easy visual tool that helps children keep track of their school items. Assign each subject a color and use that color for all related items. If you assign the color green to math, choose a green book cover, buy a green notebook, green flashcards, and a green highlighter. AD/HD children tend to be visually oriented and this visual cue is a quick and effective method to increase organization.

How do I get my child to plan ahead for projects?

Planning ahead and AD/HD do not often exist together. Planning interferes with living in the moment. Not only do AD/HD children fail to plan, they often neglect to tell their parents that they even have a project that needs planning.

If your child is assigned a book report on the first of the month and it is due on the 30th, you will need to work with her to make a list of each step necessary to complete the project. Help her transfer that list to her calendar, working backward from the due date. Use a pencil so that changes can be made along the way.

Plan how many pages she is going to read each day. If she has a 200-page book, write on her calendar "read ten pages" on each weekday and "read twenty pages" on each weekend day. Pencil in which days she will write her rough draft, edit, finalize, and type or write her final report. Be sure to use manageable goals. AD/HD children are easily overwhelmed and need to be repeatedly refocused on the small step they are working on at the moment.

How can I find out what my child's homework is?

Frequent communication with your child's teacher is the answer. Many AD/HD children hide their homework from their parents, forget to write it down, copy it incorrectly from the board, or forget to bring home their books. Expect these behaviors to be common occurrences that won't respond to punishment.

Instead of searching for the magic consequence that will work, save yourself and your child a lot of frustration and accept these behaviors as part of the disorder. Try to find creative ways to prevent them from happening in the first place.

Obtaining the entire week's assignments on either Friday or Monday, listing the homework on a website, or sending out the homework via a daily email eliminates this problem for the entire class.

If your child is fortunate enough to have her teacher use one of these methods for the class, you are in the lucky minority. Busy teachers are unlikely to have time to create a website or send out email to all parents. Busy teachers, however, might be open to parents volunteering to take on the job.

How can I get my child to use an assignment book?

Since most AD/HD children are not happy about doing homework in the first place, they lack motivation to write down their assignments. The most effective technique to combat this is to have her show her assignment book to the teacher at the end of the school day. Once the teacher checks it for accuracy, he initials it so that you know the proper information was written. For doing both of these steps, your child can earn points or tiny prizes and privileges.

If you pick your child up from school, it is a good idea to look at her assignment book before you leave the campus, providing an opportunity to run back to class if assignments were not written, signature not obtained, or books forgotten.

While most AD/HD children who do not write down their homework simply forget, be aware that children who find homework particularly tortuous may purposely "forget" and get into a pattern of lying. Use a homework website, email, or call another parent to obtain the homework to teach him that he will not escape homework by lying or forgetting to have the teacher sign the book.

Should I give my child breaks during homework?

No one answer fits every AD/HD child. If your child is able to take his break and return to the table and get back to work without delay, then a break is effective. However, if breaks cause more problems than they relieve, they should be avoided. For most AD/HD children, taking a break simply makes it more difficult to get back to their homework.

Instead of giving your child a break, you can give her a brief mental shift from homework by giving points or tiny rewards such as a sticker or a piece of candy for each set number of problems or each time period worked. These frequent rewards give your child something to be excited about and work toward. Seeing her poker chips add up or eating his candy can provide reinforcement and substitute well for breaks.

Transitioning from one activity to the next is a frequent problem for children with AD/HD. Taking a break from homework to play is no problem, of course! However, getting your child to accept that his break is over and he needs to get back to doing his homework can turn into increased procrastination, refusal to return to the table, and emotional outbursts.

Are there any devices that can aid my child in homework?

Today's children have tools available to them that parents could never dream of. The majority of AD/HD children have trouble writing neatly, making frequent erasures and producing illegible handwriting. A computer instantly solves those problems while allowing your child to demonstrate her knowledge without the added stress of the quality of her penmanship.

Creative writing is also very difficult for children with AD/HD. These children will tell you that they can "think" of what they want to say, but cannot get it down on paper. This is so pervasive as to be a legitimate problem and not just an excuse they offer up to get out of the work. Computer voice recognition software eliminates this problem like magic. Your child simply talks normally into a computer microphone and his words appear on the screen. This allows him to get his thoughts out of his head and onto paper with ease. Later, he can edit for appropriate writing style.

Books on tape and compact disc also help children who have difficulty reading. They can read along while listening, allowing them to receive the information in two forms. This can increase their skills in sight reading as well as visual and auditory comprehension.

Where should my child do homework?

Save your money and skip buying a desk for your child's room. Sending an AD/HD child to his room alone to do his homework is like sending a snail to win a race. If your AD/HD child does not need supervision to do his homework, consider both of you very lucky.

The most common and most successful location for homework is the dining room table. However, sitting at a table is not always necessary. Since AD/HD children are physically restless, they may have trouble sitting still. The table and chair setup mimics school too much for some children and the mere fact of having to sit up stimulates frustration. Many children like to stand while working, some like to roam around the room, others like to lay down, and very hyperactive children may even want to jump and roll around. As long as they can do the work, allowing physical movement is acceptable for assignments that allow for it.

Practicing spelling words, drilling mathematics, reviewing flashcards, and answering study questions are examples of homework that can be done with movement. Using creativity is key to inspiring AD/HD children to engage in tasks they are resistant to.

Are there strategies to decrease my child's homework anxiety?

The quickest way to help your child become less anxious about homework is for you to become less anxious about it. Much of your child's anxiety about homework may stem from his fear of the conflict he anticipates from you. Talk calmly and confidently to him to help him relax.

Your child will also approach homework more calmly when she knows exactly what is expected of her. AD/HD children have trouble anticipating the future. Without an exact end in sight, she may feel as if she'll be at the homework table for an eternity. Make a plan of either how much work she needs to complete or how long she needs to work.

AD/HD children are easily overwhelmed when they look at the stack of work they have to do. They begin to panic and think it will be impossible to ever finish. Their anxiety shows up disguised as avoidance, arguments, and procrastination. Clear the table of all books and materials unrelated to the assignment at hand. Anxiety can also be decreased by covering up the entire page except the row of problems he is working on at the moment.

Should I punish my child for not doing homework?

If only punishment were effective in getting AD/HD children to do their homework! For many AD/HD children, homework is so miserable that they would rather have the punishment. Parents and psychologists alike will tell you that punishment not only doesn't work in increasing compliance with homework, it actually makes the situation worse.

Common punishment strategies that parents should avoid include withholding dinner or sleep until homework is completed, making the child wake up early to finish last night's homework, using the weekend to finish work, grounding, and spanking. Teachers should avoid giving detention, denying recess and lunch time, and sending home incomplete classwork as extra homework.

These interventions may be helpful for non-AD/HD children; however, for those with AD/HD, these methods simply make the situation worse. The child can fall into a deep hole of incomplete work that he feels he can never climb out of. Homework is rapidly viewed as a burden and something to avoid at all costs. Time with family, friends, and free play is an essential part of everyone's life and depriving AD/HD children of such emotionally nurturing experiences to complete their homework only increases problems.

When should my child be able to do his own homework?

General homework guidelines do not apply to AD/HD children. Parents usually have to assist their AD/HD child for years beyond what they expect. You can save yourself a lot of angst by understanding that AD/HD has its biggest and most dramatic effect on school and homework. Expect symptoms to appear on homework days and remind yourself that they are a result of the disorder.

Instead of setting your expectations according to your child's age level, set them at his functioning level. Forget about how old he is or what grade he's in. Instead, observe what he can and cannot manage. Observe what he needs to help him with the entire homework process, from writing it down at school to returning it the next day. Give him the support he needs until he demonstrates the capacity to work more independently.

Expect that some days he will surprise you and do everything on his own, and other days it will seem like he never even heard of the word "homework." Adjust your help according to how he is functioning each day. Just because he did it yesterday, does not mean he is going to be able to do it today.

How can teachers help with homework?

Teachers want children to succeed and will usually be interested in your input as to what might be helpful for your child. A meeting at the beginning of the year with your child's teacher to enlist her help is time well spent for both you and her. Remember, teachers do not like being told how to do their job anymore than your child likes to be told to do homework. Adopt a team approach and let the teacher tell you how she intends to work with your child. Then you can contribute some ideas that you believe might help your child be successful in her class.

Some simple ways your child's teacher may be able to assist without causing extra work include:

- Announce when it is time to write down homework
- Write the assignment on the board
- Read the assignment aloud
- Provide lessons in using an assignment book
- Have an eye-catching "homework in" box clearly marked in the front of the classroom
- Announce when it is time to turn in homework
- Assign a homework monitor to collect everyone's homework
- Give a sticker, point, or token when homework is turned in
- Collect homework at roll call
- Provide lessons in using a calendar for long-term assignments

What if nothing seems to help?

When deciding if the interventions you have tried have been of any help, be sure that you have a realistic perspective of what "help" means. Of course, every parent wants to try out a new technique and have it stop the problems. If it were that simple, your child would not have a disorder. Instead, he would just be in need of some changes in your parenting. For children with AD/HD, no technique is going to "cure" the disorder or eliminate all the symptoms.

A technique "helps" if it decreases how often the problems occur. It also helps if it decreases how intense and long lasting the problem is, such as less arguing or shorter tantrums.

If everything you tried on your own is unsuccessful, it may be time to seek professional expertise. The first option is to request Section 504 accommodations and modifications for homework. During the time you are waiting for the Section 504 meeting, seek the services of a psychologist specializing in AD/HD. A psychologist can help determine causes of the problems and design interventions to prevent, decrease, and eliminate them. A tutor specializing in AD/HD can also be of great assistance with homework strategies.

How can Section 504 accommodations and modifications help with homework?

There is no reason for a child with AD/HD to suffer excessive emotional stress as the result of having to do homework. The accommodations and modifications provided by Section 504 can allow your child to do homework in a way that does not cause unreasonable psychological symptoms.

Some of the accommodations and modifications that AD/HD children may benefit from include the list below. In your Section 504 meeting, feel free to propose solutions that you think may aide your child in doing his homework.

- Cutting the quantity of homework in half
- Setting a fixed time limit for your child to work on homework
- Allowing your child to type rather than handwrite homework
- Teacher signature of homework turned in
- Providing extra time to complete projects
- Allow an extra set of textbooks to remain at home
- Assignment of a study buddy to help with assignment book
- Allow your child to correct errors for full credit
- Provide advanced warning of long term projects
- Teacher signature of assignments written in assignment book
- Prohibit the sending home of incomplete classwork as homework
- Grades will not depend on neatness
- Allow for periodic take home tests

Chapter 6

PARENTING:
RULES,
ROUTINES,
& REWARDS

- Why is structure important for AD/HD children?
- Why are rules so important for AD/HD children?
- Why is consistency so important for AD/HD children?
- What rules must I absolutely enforce?
- What are predictable consequences?
- How do I use praise to improve my child's behavior?
- How do I tell my child what I want him to do?
- Can I use a point system to improve my child's behavior?
- What rewards should my child be able to earn?
- How do I know how many points to assign each reward?
- What are the rules about the point system?
- What is the benefit of having a rulebook?
- How do I stay out of power struggles?
- What behaviors should I just give up on?
- Is spanking effective with AD/HD children?
- Can a time out be effective?
- What are the steps to giving a time-out?
- How can immediate consequences improve my child's behavior?
- How do I effectively remove privileges?
- Is a reward the same as using a bribe?
- Will rewards make my child always expect something in exchange for cooperating?
- How do I use contracts to improve my child's behavior?
- What is a parenting team?
- Should I give my child an allowance?
- What chores should I expect my child to do?
- What should I do about tantrums?
- How do I get my child to care about consequences?
- What is a good routine to set during the school week?
- What is a good routine for the weekends?
- Nothing I do makes any difference—now what do I do?

Why is structure important for AD/HD children?

Structure refers to having a predictable routine in daily life. Events happen in a certain order at a certain time. The majority of people, adults included, function better when there is structure to the day. It is anxiety provoking to wake up and not know what the day will bring. We all do better with a routine.

AD/HD children need more structure in their daily lives than most children do. Every day is like the movie *Groundhog Day* for these children. They wake up in the morning confused, having no idea what it is they are supposed to do. Every day is a brand new day. Because of their forgetfulness, it is critical that the days be structured for them. Eventually they learn the routine.

A large poster board on the bedroom wall that lists each task your child must do, in the order he should do them, can help to remind your child exactly what he needs to do each day. A picture of the task makes it easier for children who cannot read. For older children and teens, the list can be typed on regular paper and hung on a bulletin board.

Why are rules so important for AD/HD children?

Rules are important for every child and adult. They tell what is expected of us and what the consequences will be if we break those rules. Rules help us to feel comfortable that others around us will behave in appropriate ways.

AD/HD children are unfortunately frequent rule breakers, not because they don't care about the rules, but they forget the rules or cannot resist the impulse to break the rule—even if they recall what it is. Because AD/HD children lack judgment in making decisions and cannot readily determine if their actions will be acceptable, the rules need to be spelled out for every behavior. Rules also have to be spelled out in every setting, as AD/HD children do not generalize well from one situation to the next. A rule that he must keep his hands to himself when playing with his brother will not translate into keeping his hands to himself when playing with his neighbor.

You will forever be creating new rules as your child finds unique ways to misbehave that you never could have dreamed of.

Why is consistency so important for AD/HD children?

Consistency means being reliable and predictable. It is critical in the life of an AD/HD child. Not only do rules of behavior need to be clearly spelled out for the AD/HD child, they must be consistently enforced. AD/HD children are master negotiators, bringing their parents to the end of their patience with their relentless bargaining. Consistent rules eliminate the opportunity for successful bargaining and negotiations. Your child can beg, bargain, and negotiate all he wants, but the rules are the rules. The rules need to be the same day in and day out so that your child knows what to expect each time he breaks a rule.

Consistency is also needed when your child cooperates. He needs to be praised each time he is compliant. If he is on a point system, he must be able to count on you to give him his points, privileges, and rewards, otherwise he will quickly lose motivation.

Parents also need consistency. Never knowing what surprise behavior your child will engage in from day to day, you need to know that you can at least stick to the routine. Consistency in rules and consequences also ensures that you do not have to decide each day what rules to enforce and what consequences to give.

What rules must I absolutely enforce?

Each parent has certain behaviors he or she will not tolerate as well as ones they are not concerned with. Some parents will not tolerate talking back while others cannot accept a messy room. Because AD/HD children engage in so many inappropriate behaviors, it is impossible to set a consequence for them all. Even if you tried, you would be unable to point out to your child each of his misbehaviors. Sometimes your child will be simultaneously engaging in so many inappropriate actions that you won't know which one to tell him to stop.

Instead, you must determine which behaviors and tasks you believe are the most important. You have to choose your battles. It is easier to first make a list of which behaviors and tasks you can let go. A clean room should be on the top of the list of behaviors to give up.

The list of behaviors that all children should do includes brushing teeth, bathing, going to school, and doing some homework. Behaviors that all children should be disciplined for include physical violence, property destruction, cursing, and threats of violence.

What are predictable consequences?

It is a daunting prospect to attempt to create a consequence for all the problem behaviors your AD/HD child engages in. Even if you could write a rule for every misdeed, it's unrealistic to think that you would have the time, patience, and stamina to develop consequences for each one. Fortunately, by using predictable consequences, you don't have to.

Predictable consequences are the automatic results of behavior that occur without you having to do anything. A child who refuses to eat dinner will go hungry. If your son refuses to wear his jacket to school, he will be cold. If he throws his toy in anger and breaks it, he no longer has the pleasure of that toy. These are situations where the punishment simply presents itself. Parents do not have to be the punisher in situations that have a predictable consequence. Instead, they can be an empathic parent who calmly says, "That's what happens, honey, when you don't take an umbrella, you get rained on. Next time maybe you'll make a better choice." Nature doled out the punishment and you can save your discipline for situations when there is not a predictable consequence.

How do I use praise to improve my child's behavior?

Despite appearances, most AD/HD children really do want to do what is right. They are very responsive to praise and, if they know it is readily available, they will work to earn it.

Praise is the easiest parenting technique to use, but also the easiest to forget. It is difficult to find the compassion to praise behaviors that parents of nondisordered children simply come to expect. AD/HD children, however, need to be recognized for the most basic of behaviors.

Praise needs to be given frequently, enthusiastically, and sincerely. The more often you catch your child behaving appropriately, the more opportunity he has to feel good about himself. It is with incessant praise that small behaviors will eventually become part of your child's daily repertoire. Having the confidence to perform one behavior provides the strength for your child to tackle another.

Look for opportunities to praise your child. Give praise with a smile, hug, or pat of affection. When praising, resist the temptation to turn it into a lesson for inappropriate behavior. It is not praise if you follow a compliment with "Why can't you always do that?!"

How do I tell my child what I want him to do?

The use of commands will increase the chances that your child will do what you tell him to do. The language of commands makes it clear that you expect cooperation. A command is not a request. You do not ask your child if he would like to brush his teeth, you give him a command that it is "time to brush your teeth."

In giving a command, you must first decide that the behavior needs to be done and it is not something you can let go or ignore. You need to have a consequence in mind to use if he does not comply. Then you must decide if you are willing to follow through to the end. If not, do not give the command.

Put your command in a positive direction, telling your child exactly what to do. "Take your feet off the coffee table" may result in the feet ending up on the couch. A more direct command is to say, "Put your feet on the floor please." An immediate "thank you" will increase future cooperation.

Can I use a point system to improve my child's behavior?

A well-organized point system can result in dramatic improvement in your child's behavior. A weekly chart of all the tasks your child must do, alongside a row for each day of the week is an easy way to keep track of what points were earned. The chart is also the best way to monitor which tasks are being consistently completed and which ones are areas of conflict.

One point per task or behavior makes the point system simple and easier for parents and children to follow. Equal point value also helps to ensure that children will not pick and choose which behaviors they will do based upon the amount of points. Points are totaled at the end of the evening. Bedtime is a nice time to snuggle with your child while reviewing her chart. Talk enthusiastically to your child about all the behaviors they earned points for. Give your child encouragement that tomorrow is a new day and she can try to earn points for the behaviors she missed today.

Each day your child will be able to cash in points for a wide variety of items, treats, and privileges.

What rewards should my child be able to earn?

In order to make the point system exciting and motivating for your child, you need to have a variety of rewards and privileges for her to choose from. Ask your child to help you make a list of desired activities, food treats, and items to buy. While some rewards will entail money, the majority of rewards should be free or very low cost. Regardless of your income, rewards are to motivate, not to overindulge.

Fun activities can be considered rewards. Despite children believing that the use of television, computers, and video games are rights, they are actually privileges earned by good behavior. An AD/HD child's love of these activities can be worked to your advantage. Assign ten points per half hour for these activities. Besides reading a book and playing with their toys, all other activities need to be paid for with points.

Special food treats can be powerful motivators. Small items of gum, candy, and an occasional soda can excite children to earn their points. Larger treats of pizza, dessert, or choosing where the family goes to dinner can be bigger rewards.

Items that your child asks for should be added to his reward list instead of merely bought for them.

How do I know how many points to assign each reward?

You want your child to earn and spend points easily. The idea is to provide a rewarding environment that shows your child numerous times each day that if he behaves well, he will be rewarded.

A general guideline is to have enough small privileges, treats, and items so that your child can spend some of his points every day, yet have enough opportunity to earn points that he can bank some to save for bigger rewards.

Activities of television, video games, and computer time can be assigned ten points per half hour. Playing outside is free unless he wants to ride bikes or rollerblade outside the home. In that case, ten points per half hour would be considered reasonable. Renting a DVD is thirty points, a sleepover is fifty points, and going to the movies is one hundred points.

Food treats should be easy to spend points on. Five points per gum, candy, or cookie gives your child a desirable reward he can easily earn. Bigger treats of pizza, fast food, or choosing where the family eats dinner should cost one hundred points. Items your child wants to buy should be charged according to their expense. A general guideline is to charge fifty points for every dollar. You might want your child to engage in some behaviors without having to pay points. Which events are free will vary from family to family. A general guideline is to not charge points for activities that you want to encourage. Special outings with the family, religious activities, extracurricular activities, and walking with parents after dinner each night are examples of activities you may want to make "free." Occasional events where you have advance warning, such as a friend's birthday party or a sleepover, can be great motivators for your child to earn enough points to be able to attend. Assign a point value that you absolutely know your child can earn specifically for the special event.

What are the rules about the point system?

It is important to specify the rules ahead of time. Points must be spent within the family rules. A child cannot spend his one hundred points on ten straight hours of television or twenty sodas. Your daughter cannot spend points on a sleepover if she was suspended from school.

Parents need to find a balance between making rewards available and keeping rules. Changes in your child's behavior have to occur alongside changes in your attitude about rewards. Most parents do not like their child to watch excessive television. Children, on the other hand, love television. If knowing she can watch her favorite TV show once she has finished her homework motivates your child to get to work and not argue with you, maybe television is not worth withholding. The same holds true for food treats. No parent likes her child to have sugar every day. Yet, if bath time gets done calmly with the anticipation of spending points on a treat, maybe a scoop of ice cream each night is not so bad.

Parents need to make compromises in rewards in exchange for improved behavior. Peace in the household can be more important than being strict on certain privileges.

What is the benefit of having a rulebook?

A rulebook provides parents and children the chance to work together to make decisions, in advance, about what behaviors are expected and what consequences will occur if a rule is broken. Determining consequences ahead of the misbehavior is advantageous for both parents and child.

With the rulebook, children know exactly what is expected of them and what will occur if they do not meet that expectation. This removes the guessing game for the child of wondering whether he will be in trouble for his misdeeds. He knows in advance what his consequence will be.

For parents, the rulebook reminds them of the expectations and consequences they deem appropriate when misbehavior occurs. This makes parenting easier by removing the problem of having to think on your feet of what consequence to give. It also prevents you from being too mild when you are in a particularly good mood or too harsh when you are losing your patience.

When arguments begin over punishment being "unfair" or "different" from last time, parents merely have to direct their child to the rulebook. Couples can refer to the rulebook when one begins to deviate from the agreed upon consequences.

How do I stay out of power struggles?

AD/HD children, especially those who have coexisting ODD, are very skilled at pulling parents into power struggles. The strongest parent can easily find themselves in the midst of arguments and negotiations.

The best way to stay out of a power struggle is to not enter it in the first place. Do not set a limit or make a demand unless you are prepared to follow through and make it happen.

Children are quite astute at observing your behavior and quickly figuring out when you mean business.

Understanding your child's motivation for a power struggle helps you to remain detached during the argument. As long as your child can keep you arguing, he escapes having to comply. While it makes no sense to parents why their child would choose a drawn out battle over simply doing the task that could be over in minutes, for the AD/HD child, the only thing that matters is "right now this very second." If he can avoid complying for the moment, in his mind he is winning. He can't see the overall picture. While he wins for the moment, he loses a lot of time in the conflict and will ultimately have to comply anyway.

What behaviors should I just give up on?

It is okay to discard certain behaviors and tasks from your expectations of your child. Customize what you ask of your child to be consistent with his functioning level. Asking your ten-year-old AD/HD child to perform the same chores and responsibilities of a nondisordered ten-year-old is a certain formula for constant family upset.

Give up making demands on your child that you cannot enforce. There are certain behaviors that you absolutely cannot make your child do. You cannot make them stop crying, eat, stop talking, and go to sleep. Insisting your child stop crying only demonstrates your inability to have authority over your child. Make requests and set limits that you can make happen.

Give up on chores that cause daily arguments. Do not expect your child to make his bed, clean his room, and feed the dog. These simply won't happen on any regular basis, even with nondisordered children. Focus on the tasks that are important to complete.

AD/HD children give their parents plenty of opportunity to nag, cajole, threaten, yell, lecture, and punish. You can make life more pleasant for you and your child by eliminating many of the unnecessary tasks.

Is spanking effective with AD/HD children?

Spanking has been found, for all children, to have many more negative results than positive changes. Physical aggression is simply not necessary in order to teach or punish any child.

Some parents say spanking does work, yet you would be hard-pressed to find a parent of an AD/HD child that would tell you spanking stopped the problem behaviors. If spanking could change a child's behavior, it would be because the AD/HD child was able to think ahead and stop his impulsive and inappropriate behavior. This would mean that he took the time to reflect back on how last time he did the same behavior he was spanked. It would also mean that he was able to anticipate the consequence by recalling that spankings hurt. Since he does not want to hurt, he will not misbehave. If the AD/HD child could use this type of thinking, he wouldn't need any punishment and he would not have AD/HD!

Instead of stopping the inappropriate behavior, spanking often results in anger and resentment toward parents. Rest assured, after a spanking, your child is not thinking about what he did wrong. He is instead thinking about how mad he is at you. If he has coexisting ODD, he is also thinking about how he will get revenge.

Can a time-out be effective?

Time-out is the behavior modification technique of giving the child "time away" from any positive reinforcement. It is a highly effective technique in stopping inappropriate behavior in its tracks. Some parents might say it doesn't work; however, their expectations are that if they give a few time-outs, it should stop the problem behavior completely.

Time-out for AD/HD children is a management technique, not a cure. With proper understanding that it is intended to stop behavior in the present and prevent it for a brief period of time afterward, you will find the usefulness of a time-out.

The idea of time-out is to make the time in the chair unrewarding. The command to go to time-out should be brief and direct and not involve any discussion. While the child is in the chair, there is no contact with her. After the time-out is over, there is no lecture, discussion, or affection. Your child simply goes back to her activity or, if she was requested to do a task, she must now do the task that caused the time-out. Conducting time-out this way ensures that you don't make the aftermath a rewarding experience.

What are the steps to giving a time-out?

Place a chair away from all stimulation. A hallway, entry way, or kitchen is a good location. Your chair need not be solely for time-out.

Give your child a chance to comply with a request to either stop a behavior or do a task. A second request is made if he has not complied, this time with the warning that if he does not comply he will have a time-out. If you have to ask a third time, you say, "You did not do as I asked, you now have a time-out."

When your child sits in the chair, you set a timer that he can see. One minute per year of age is a general guideline for AD/HD children. Time-out is over when the timer goes off.

If your child refuses to go to time-out, give a warning that if he chooses not to go, you will take him there and his time in the chair will double. If he is small, you can physically take him there. If he is too big for you to safely manage, you must not enter into a physical power struggle. Instead, withhold all rewards and privileges until he takes his time-out.

How can immediate consequences improve my child's behavior?

Immediate is the name of the game for AD/HD children. They live in the immediate moment. The only time that matters is right now. These children do not look back and they don't look forward.

Praise and punishment for AD/HD children both work best if they are done immediately after a behavior. Praise helps your child feel good about himself right after he has done well.

Punishment is also more effective if it is given as close to the misbehavior as possible. It should be swift and last only for a short time. Loss of a favorite toy or activity should start as soon as the behavior is reprimanded and last until the next morning. Grounding from all privileges follows the same timeline.

Short-term consequences give the child hope and motivation to do well the next day. If he is grounded for one week, what is his incentive to behave for the rest of the week? You can be sure that he will do something that warrants grounding and, if already grounded, he has no motivation to cooperate.

How do I effectively remove privileges?

In the nondisordered world of parenting, you say "no computer until tomorrow" and your child does not use the computer until tomorrow. In the AD/HD and ODD world, you say "no computer until tomorrow" and your child uses the computer the minute you leave her room.

Be prepared to be tough and enforce your removal of privileges. Before you remove a privilege, you should state the request and wait for compliance. A second request follows continued noncompliance with a warning: "If you choose not to turn off the video now, you will lose the use of it until tomorrow." If your child does not turn it off, you must do so. You cannot let him rope you into a battle over who is in charge. If he won't cooperate with you, take charge and turn it off.

If he is prone to use the video despite being grounded from it, you take charge and remove it from his room. Inform him that you are "taking your video out of your room until tomorrow because the last time you lost this privilege you played video games anyway. Until I can trust you, I will keep it when you lose your privilege."

Is a reward the same as using a bribe?

Some parents wonder if they reward their child for good behavior, are they bribing them. A reward is not a bribe. A bribe is giving something in exchange for immoral or illegal behavior. A reward is a legal and moral reinforcement in exchange for good behavior.

The structure of our society works on rewards. While going to work may not seem rewarding, if you work you are rewarded with a paycheck. We are given money in exchange for good work. We change that money in for our most basic rewards of food, clothing, and shelter. With extra money, we reward ourselves with less necessary but satisfying objects and experiences. If you did not receive a paycheck, how long would you keep showing up to your job?

Children need to be rewarded for their work too. Their job is to cooperate with their parents, do their best in school, and learn to become a good member of society. Some children have this drive in them naturally. Many AD/HD children, however, are lacking an internal motivation to behave just because that is the proper thing to do. Many need an external reason to try hard. Rewards provide that incentive and are very effective.

Will rewards make my child always expect something in exchange for cooperating?

When first starting a point system, it is common that for every request you make of your child, she will ask you if she is going to earn points or a prize if she complies. Parents mistakenly see this as a sign that their child will never again cooperate without promise of a prize.

This behavior is actually a positive sign and can be used to your advantage. You want her to ask about her points and how she can earn them. You want her to be thinking about the point system, her behavior, and earning prizes for being good. By asking, she demonstrates that she is thinking about her choices regarding her behavior. True, she is weighing the pros and cons of cooperating, but at least she is stopping to calculate her decision.

The eventual goal is for her to cooperate because that is the right thing to do. In years to come, slowly and eventually she will develop an internal drive to do what is requested without reward. Until that time comes, let her ask about her points and encourage her to cooperate to earn them.

How do I use contracts to improve my child's behavior?

Most AD/HD children have a higher-than-normal drive to earn rewards and privileges. Their incessant hunger for playing video games, collecting trading cards, and using the computer allows parents to offer powerful rewards in exchange for cooperation.

Verbal contracts guarantee endless arguments that your child will not easily back down from. Signed, written contracts, however, remove all chances for your child to successfully argue his way into a bigger reward. Both parent and child sign and date the contract so that when your child later argues, and he will, you can direct him to read the contract.

You can make as many contracts as you both agree to; however, they must have only one behavior and one reward per contract. Behaviors and rewards must be specific. Contracting for playing video games if your child is "good for one week" does not tell your child exactly what "good" means or how long he gets to play the video game. Instead, contract for your child to have no time-outs all day in exchange for one hour of video games starting after dinner.

Due to the AD/HD child's difficulty delaying gratification, contracts should be short-term.

What is a parenting team?

Raising a child is one of the most challenging endeavors any adult can have. It is also one of the most trying aspects of marriage. Research has shown for decades that marital satisfaction is at its lowest during the eighteen years it takes to raise a child. If the marriage can survive, and fewer than 50 percent do, marital happiness returns to pre-child levels.

Add to this statistic the challenge of raising an AD/HD child! Many couples with an AD/HD child report frequent disagreements and arguments over the rearing of their child. Mothers tend to be inconsistent in their discipline, while fathers often deny that their child has a disorder. The child is raised in an unpredictable environment and quickly learns how to manipulate both parents.

If parents hope to keep a steady relationship and have consistency in the household, they must work together as a team. This means having meetings to discuss what your child's behavioral difficulties are and mapping out a discipline plan that you both will use to manage the troubles. Teamwork means frequent and open communication and compromise. Both parents must be working from the same rulebook, point system, and contracts.

Should I give my child an allowance?

An allowance can be a strong motivator for children to cooperate and complete their tasks. Children should earn their allowance, not simply be given money.

For AD/HD children, an allowance must be carefully designed. The nondisordered child can earn a fixed allowance if they have a good week and do all their tasks. The AD/HD child would never earn his allowance based on this design!

Structuring an allowance for the AD/HD child is best done incrementally. Your child can earn small sums for small tasks. The more tasks he completes, the more money he earns. This sets up the allowance program to be successful. No matter how bad a week your child had, he is bound to have done a few things that earned some allowance.

Ask your child what tasks he would like to do in exchange for allowance. If he selects some of the tasks, he will be more motivated to complete them than if you tell him everything he must do. Assign each task a monetary value, with easy tasks earning less money and more difficult tasks earning more money. Regardless of your financial ability, it is important that the allowance is reasonable and teaches the value of working for money.

What chores should I expect my child to do?

All children should complete some chores. Which ones will depend not so much on your child's age, but more on his ability. Additional chores can be added as you see your child is capable.

Picking up toys is probably the first chore your child will have starting in her toddler years. As your child progresses, she can begin to put away her clothes and hang up her bath towel. These are likely to be the only chores your child does until mid-elementary school years. You will have to remind and directly supervise your AD/HD child during these chores for far longer than you think. Give up the expectation that she will remember to do these on her own and will do it with you asking only one time.

By fourth grade, your child should be able to add a small chore of taking out the trash, setting or clearing the table, or putting away the laundry. Surprisingly, many AD/HD children enjoy vacuuming and dusting and want to add it to their allowance list. Middle school and high school years can add a daily chore such as doing the dishes, laundry, or cleaning the bathroom.

What should I do about tantrums?

Toddlers are expected to have tantrums. By age four, they should have gained skills in accepting the disappointment of not getting what they want. Some AD/HD children, however, throw tantrums long past their toddler years.

Some AD/HD children will hit their parents, throw objects, punch holes in walls, and purposely break things. Minor upsets of having to turn off the television can provoke a rage far out of proportion.

You cannot make your child stop his tantrum. Therefore, tantrum-throwing children should be sent to time-out until their tantrum is over. Small children can be physically placed in the time-out chair, but bigger children can start a physical brawl that can be dangerous to both themselves and their parent. These children should be directed to go their room where they may finish their tantrum. Many children will comply with this command, but then they will destroy their room. Parents need to make sure their child is physically safe in the room and that there are no dangerous objects they can harm themselves with. The child should then be left alone to work himself out of the tantrum. As a consequence, whatever damage he caused, he must later clean up and pay for.

How do I get my child to care about consequences?

The idea of removing a privilege is to have your child upset enough by its loss that he will think twice before he repeats the same misbehavior. After all, that is the whole idea behind this parenting tool.

Some parents of AD/HD children find it very difficult to find a privilege to remove that has an effect on their child. Their child will throw a tantrum if he has to turn off the television to go to bed, but when he loses his computer for one week, he may shrug it off and continue his misbehavior as if he were never punished. Their child's failure to show distress leads some parents to abandon this technique.

Consequences still need to be given, regardless of your child's reaction. Even if he is not showing distress, he is still missing the opportunity to have his favorite item or activity. He may truly not care and can easily move onto another activity, or he may be upset but clever enough to hide it from you in an attempt to make you drop this punishment in the future.

What is a good routine to set during the school week?

Your child should have a set time to wake up each school day. AD/HD children are often quite irritable in the morning and do not wake up easily. Time to wake up before getting out of bed should be built into the schedule for these children. To increase cooperation, your child can help select the order in which he wants to list the tasks on his chart. All tasks, no matter how minor, should be listed. Using the toilet, brushing teeth, dressing in school clothes, putting on shoes, putting pajamas away, eating breakfast, putting lunch in his backpack, and taking his backpack to school are typical morning routine tasks. Having the list can decrease the number of reminders parents have to give. Children can be redirected to check their chart if they forget their next task.

The after-school routine can include a snack and a brief period of relaxation before homework. Free time should begin only after homework is completed. A regular family dinner hour followed by helping with the dishes builds in family time and an opportunity to be helpful. Bath followed by free time until bedtime ensures that responsibilities are completed before free time occurs.

What is a good routine for the weekends?

While AD/HD children need routine, they also need unstructured time. Being free to play is as important as completing required tasks. Weekend activities will vary from family to family and from weekend to weekend. While the weekends may mean complete freedom for some, many children are active in sports, religious activities, social events, and hobbies on Saturdays. Chores, homework, book reports, and school projects often take place on the weekend as well. For what is supposed to be unstructured free time, the weekends of many children are booked solid with activities. It is important to try to find a balance between structured activities and free time.

Free time provides your child with a chance to simply play without structure, rules, or having to please anyone or achieve a particular goal or purpose.

In addition to your child simply having free time on his own, it is also important to make time on the weekend for the family to have fun. You and your child can enjoy one another's company without the stresses of the weekdays.

Nothing I do makes any difference—now what do I do?

This feeling is more common than not in parents of AD/HD children. No matter what you try, nothing seems to make any lasting difference. There is a good reason for this.

Nothing you do as a parent will cure the disorder. The behaviors that your AD/HD child exhibits will be with her throughout her childhood. You will be far less frustrated if you understand that parenting techniques are designed to manage the symptoms of AD/HD by decreasing their frequency, intensity, and severity, not to cure them.

AD/HD children are not your average children and they do not readily respond to the usual parenting methods. Parents raising AD/HD children need to go above and beyond the usual parenting techniques. Be sure your parenting skills include:

- Creating a rulebook
- Structuring your child's life
- Working as a parenting team
- Designing and using a point system
- Frequently praising
- Giving immediate consequences
- Using time-out

If life in your house is not more manageable after you have tried these techniques, then it is time to seek assistance. A child psychologist can work with you to teach you where changes need to be made. Once life is stable at home, periodic visits to the psychologist can help keep your parenting in sync with your child's changes and development.

Chapter 7 — MEDICATION

- Should I medicate my child?
- Is medication being overprescribed?
- Why is medication use on the rise?
- Which children are most likely to be prescribed medication?
- What is the controversy about medication?
- What can medication do to help?
- Will medication stop all the symptoms?
- Is medication alone enough?
- Does medication improve a child's ability to learn?
- What types of medication are used to treat AD/HD?
- How do stimulant medications work?
- What are the side effects of stimulant medication?
- How are the side effects of stimulant medication managed?
- Can stimulant medication cause tics?
- What is sustained release medication?
- What are the types of nonstimulant medications used?
- What are the side effects of nonstimulant medication?
- Is medication necessary on nonschool days?
- Is the medication addictive?
- Does stimulant medication lead to later drug use?
- What are the long-term effects of medication?
- How long will my child have to take medication?
- How do children feel about taking medication?
- What do I do if my child refuses to take medications?
- Does medication teach children that they need pills to succeed?
- How do parents feel about giving their child medication?
- What factors should I consider before giving my child medication?
- Will I experience pressure to medicate my child?
- How do I resist pressure to give my child medication?

Should I medicate my child?

The decision to give your child psychiatric medication is a highly personal one; one that should be made only after a thorough evaluation, in-depth consultation with the prescribing physician, and a chance to educate yourself about the various medications and non-medication treatment options. You must make the time to become an informed consumer, as medication is almost always the first option presented, and in many cases the only option.

There are pros and cons of medication. It is a game of balancing benefits with side effects and determining if the positive results outweigh the negative side effects. Only you can decide which way the scales balance.

Be prepared to hear from teachers, parents, and physicians that you absolutely should medicate your child. You will hear that over 70 percent of children taking medication receive positive benefits. Parents will tell you that medication made their child a completely different person. You will hear praises of medication that will make you wish you put it in your child's baby bottle!

Despite the praise medication receives, you must know from the beginning that medication is not a cure. Nor is it a miracle. It is a tool that helps some children with some of the symptoms, some of the time.

Is medication being overprescribed?

There is no doubt that far more prescriptions are being written in the past fifteen years than in the years previous.

Rates of stimulant medication consumption provided by the International Narcotics Control Board reveal an overall increase of 87 percent in Denmark, France, the Netherlands, New Zealand, Spain, Sweden, and the United Kingdom when usage during 1994 to 1997 was compared to usage during 1998 to 2000.

During this same period, the increase was 45 percent in the United States and 93 percent in Canada. While the increase was less in the U.S., it is still the largest consumer of stimulant medications, consuming approximately 85 percent of the world's methylphenidate. Canada is the world's second largest consumer, followed by Australia and New Zealand.

The Drug Enforcement Agency (DEA) has observed a dramatic increase in stimulants between 1991 and 1999. Amphetamine production increased more than 2,000 percent, and methylphenidate nearly 500 percent. These medications are prescribed with great variability across the U.S., with some states using three to five times the amount of other states.

Why is medication use on the rise?

Sixty to eighty percent of children in the U.S. diagnosed with AD/HD have been treated at some point with medication. Almost 30 percent of these children are treated with two or more psychiatric medications.

A variety of factors has likely contributed to the dramatic increase in stimulant use. Changes in the diagnostic criteria over the years allows for more children and teens to qualify for the diagnosis. Research findings that AD/HD often extends into adolescence have dissolved the practice of terminating medications at puberty. Long-term studies discovering that many individuals continue to have the disorder well past reaching adulthood have added a population of adults who had stopped medication as minors.

Development of longer-lasting, more effective medications with easier administration and fewer side effects increases the likelihood that individuals will take medication over longer periods of time. Physicians' comfort with prescribing medication to younger children further adds to the increase. In the 1990s, there was a three-fold increase in the number of preschool children taking stimulants despite most not being approved for those less than six years of age.

Increased public awareness and education of parents, teachers, mental health professionals, and physicians adds to the number of individuals referring children and teens for medication.

Which children are most likely to be prescribed medication?

Having a diagnosis of AD/HD more often than not results in a prescription of medication. The vast majority of all prescriptions for amphetamine and methylphenidate—about 80 percent—are written for children diagnosed with AD/HD. A variety of factors adds to the chances of a child being prescribed medication, including gender, age, income, and race.

- Caucasian children are more likely to be prescribed stimulants than African American children are.
- Boys are still prescribed stimulants more often than girls are, at a rate of about to 3:1 to 4:1, although the number of prescriptions for girls is on the increase.
- Children ages nine and ten have the highest use rate; however, both younger children and teens are increasing their use.
- Toddlers prescribed psychiatric medications are on the rise. In the year 2000, approximately 1 to 1.5 percent of children aged two to four years were receiving stimulants, antidepressants, or antipsychotic medications.
- Children from higher income families and areas that are more affluent have higher prescription rates than lower income families from less economically advantaged neighborhoods. Those who are uninsured are less likely to receive a prescription than insured children.

- Interestingly, children who have three or more siblings are less likely to receive stimulant medication.

What is the controversy about medication?

No AD/HD topic raises more emotions than prescribing stimulant medication to children. Medical doctors offer it after they make a rapid diagnosis. Teachers urge parents that medication is the only way the child will not fail the school year. Parents who have medicated their child tell you it is the only way to go. Rare is the professional or parent who urges you to try other methods first. Even more rare is the parent who absolutely refuses to give medications no matter what.

Why the push for medication? Why not urge for parent training, specialized classrooms, and social skills training? While there is no answer to this, we can hypothesize why parents are pressured to give their children medication. Medication is relatively inexpensive for parents to buy and highly profitable for pharmaceutical companies to manufacture. Medication is easy to give and takes almost no effort for parents. Keeping a child calm in the classroom is far easier with medication than behavior modification.

American culture is very comfortable with medication. Television and magazines are filled with advertisements for medication for anything that ails us. We are a very busy society that more typically has two working parents or a single parent home, leaving little time for parenting after a long day at work. With more than 50 percent of the families divorced, parents feel guilty and do not want firm discipline to upset their already emotionally scarred child. Rarely does a child today get a spanking, a positive change for decreasing child abuse, but parents have not substituted with learning effective parenting skills.

All these factors likely contribute to the ease with which our society is willing to medicate children of all ages. Parenting any child is an incredibly challenging and often frustrating task. No one ever said it would be easy. Add to the challenge the monumental job of raising an AD/HD child. If a pill can make your job easier, many parents think, "why not?" Few ever ask, "Why?" or "what can I do instead?"

Deciding whether or not to medicate should be a decision that you make only after you have carefully studied the pros and cons of medication and have determined if you have exhausted all other avenues.

What can medication do to help?

Stimulant medication has been proven time and again to have positive short-term effects. These medications can temporarily improve hyperactivity, impulsivity, and inattention. Increases in the ability to produce work, remain free from distraction, and decrease aggression have been established in the scientific research.

Research shows that 70 percent of children treated with stimulant medication show some improvement with the greatest benefits seen in the child's ability to maintain attention, concentration, and focus. Increases in these skills may in turn decrease a child's disruption of his class, increase the amount of class work and homework he completes, and allow him to sit quieter in his seat. Legibility of handwriting has repeatedly been found after taking medication. Impulsivity may decrease, resulting in fewer inappropriate behaviors. At home, a medicated child may be less restless and overactive, and better able to follow instructions and complete tasks.

It is important to know that despite the observable short-term improvements in behavior, stimulant medications do not appear to achieve long-term changes in outcomes such as peer relationships, social or academic skills, or school achievement. The benefits are quite short-term and only present while the medication is active in the body. Once the medication wears off, the benefits disappear.

Will medication stop all the symptoms?

The answer to this question is an irrefutable "no." Medication will not stop any of the symptoms. It can, however, result in a temporary cessation or decrease in problematic behaviors resulting from the core symptoms of hyperactivity, impulsivity, and inattention.

Despite potential improvements in major AD/HD symptoms, medication does little to decrease many of the related symptoms that often coexist with the disorder. Many of these additional behaviors can be more troublesome for both you and your child than inattention, overactivity, and impulsivity. Symptoms of difficulty being satisfied, tolerating frustration, playing cooperatively, sharing toys, having tantrums, and being bossy, among others, show little or no response to medication.

Medication also will not make your child a different person. It does not change personality, intelligence, or temperament. To achieve the greatest benefits from medication, your child must live in a highly structured environment. A medicated child in a home without rules, structure, predictability, and effective parenting will not function better simply because he is taking medication.

Symptoms improved by medication are done so only temporarily. Positive benefits from medication do not last after medication treatment is terminated. This is in contrast to the lasting effects of behavioral treatment.

Is medication alone enough?

The largest study of ADHD children ever conducted (MTA study) found that children who were treated with combined therapies had better results than those treated solely with medication. Medication is more effective than behavior therapy in decreasing hyperactivity, impulsivity, and distractibility. However, symptoms of aggression, defiance, and poor social skills were more responsive to a combined treatment of behavior therapy and medication.

In the MTA study, parents whose children received only medication tended to drop out of treatment and report less satisfaction than those who received a combination of behavioral and medication treatment. Behavioral treatment also provided longer-lasting results than medication alone one year after treatment was completed. In fact, after one year after treatment, the positive results achieved from medication had diminished somewhat while the benefits from behavior modification continued to remain.

The MTA study also found that while medication helped some of the primary symptoms of ADHD, medication alone was not shown to be effective for academic achievement, parent-child relations, oppositional behavior, reading, and social skills. Children who received medication combined with behavioral therapy showed more improvement in these areas than those who had medication alone.

The American Academy of Pediatrics supports combined treatment and advises pediatricians to avoid recommending medication treatment only.

Does medication improve a child's ability to learn?

Many parents choose to give medication in the hope that it will improve their child's ability to learn in school. This thought is logical and, in fact, is supported by years of research that demonstrates medication does improve school performance. While this is good news, improved performance in school does not translate into increased learning. How much a child has learned is measured each school year by standardized academic achievement tests.

Medication does not make a child learn more than he would otherwise learn without medication. Medication can improve your child's ability to produce work at school and at home. Children who are medicated can pay more attention, concentrate better, resist distraction, and remain more on task. They are able to complete more school and homework and may earn higher grades when medicated. Yet, even with these benefits, medication has not been proven by research to improve children's academic achievement on standardized testing, meaning they do not show increases in learning.

The medication may have smoothed the bumps along the road during the school year, making it easier for the child to complete his work, but he does not learn more than if he were not medicated. These consistent findings indicate that medication should not be given for the purposes of "making the child learn."

What types of medication are used to treat AD/HD?

Stimulant medication is the most commonly prescribed medication for both ADD and ADHD. Stimulants used for AD/HD include amphetamine or methylphenidate. These medications have been used for over six decades to treat behavior problems in children. Most stimulant medications are approved for children age six or older.

Stimulants are prescribed in short-acting, intermediate, and long-acting forms. Short-acting forms are taken in divided doses, usually two to three times daily, and last from three to five hours. Intermediate-acting stimulants are taken once or twice a day and last between three and eight hours. Long-acting medications are sustained release stimulants that are taken once daily and last from eight to twelve hours.

Short-acting stimulants include:
- Dexedrine
- Dextrostat
- Focalin
- Ritalin
- Methylin

Intermediate-acting stimulants include:
- Ritalin SR
- Metadate ER
- Methylin ER
- Adderall
- Dexedrine Spansule

Long-acting stimulants include:
- Concerta
- Metadate CD
- Ritalin LA
- Adderall XR

There is no way to predict which medication will be best for your child. It is a process of trial and error, trying different medications, doses, and administration times until you find the right type, amount, and schedule.

How do stimulant medications work?

While scientists do not know exactly how stimulants work, it is believed they increase the activity of chemicals, called neurotransmitters, in the parts of the brain responsible for inhibiting behavior and increasing attention. Dopamine and norepinephrine are the two neurotransmitters thought to have a significant influence on our ability to maintain focus on tasks, thus increasing attention and concentration, and to inhibit our behavior, thus decreasing restlessness and excessive physical activity.

Stimulants are taken by mouth and are quickly absorbed into the bloodstream. They are short acting and must be taken several times each day to maintain effectiveness. Many children will respond to stimulants within as little as thirty minutes. The peak time of effectiveness is during the first hour to three hours after ingestion. Positive effects last for approximately four hours. Within twenty-four hours, stimulants are excreted out of the body.

Beware of myths about how medication works. The idea that you "prove" the diagnosis by seeing if a child responds well to stimulant medication is false. In fact, medication is never used to make or verify a diagnosis. Also incorrect is the belief that stimulants have a "reverse" effect on people with AD/HD, slowing them down instead of speeding them up. For almost any person, stimulant medication will result in increased attention and concentration, along with decreased distractibility and activity.

What are the side effects of stimulant medication?

The most common side effects are transient decreased appetite, insomnia, anxiety, irritability, stomachaches, and headaches. It is quite common for children to experience one or more of these side effects in the first few weeks of treatment. Many children adapt to the medication and majority of the side effects will disappear.

Yet, for some children, decreased appetite and/or insomnia do not go away regardless of how long the child has been taking the medication. It is not unusual for some children to skip their lunch and eat large amounts of food when the medication wears off in the afternoon. Insomnia may keep children up long past their bedtime. Despite wanting to sleep, some children simply are unable to fall asleep until late into the night.

Afternoon "rebound" may be seen when the lunchtime dose wears off and the child becomes quite irritable and/or sad and tearful in the afternoon. When children have too high a dose, they may become overly focused and dull or "zombie-like."

There is no way to determine how any child will respond to medication. Trial and error is the only method to find the right dose of the right medication with the least amount of side effects.

Rare side effects of agitation, psychosis, and depression have been known to occur in some children taking stimulant medication. Recent reports of serious psychiatric symptoms in children taking methylphenidate prompted the Food and Drug Administration in June 2005 to announce that it plans to strengthen the warning labels on all methylphenidate medications. Increased reports of suicidal thoughts, hallucinations, and violent behavior in children taking methylphenidate are causing the FDA to take a closer look at these medications.

How are the side effects of stimulant medication managed?

Your child's physician is the best source for managing side effects. Modifying the dose and time of the medication is the easiest method of decreasing or eliminating side effects. Expect your child's physician to make several changes in the medication plan until she is able to find the optimum balance between positive effects and minimal side effects. These changes do not mean the doctor is experimenting with your child; it is merely part of the necessary process to find the right medication protocol.

Children who lose their appetite during the day can easily make up the calories and nutrition by making food available to them when they are hungry. Giving medication with or after breakfast and lunch can ensure adequate food intake before the medication suppresses their appetite. Insomnia can be managed by eliminating an afternoon dose of medication or giving it earlier in the day. Afternoon rebound can be offset by a minimal afternoon dose or use of sustained release medication.

A daily log showing the time medication was given, the time side effects appeared, and a rating of your child's behavior, work produced, and level of activity will allow your physician to closely evaluate if the medication type, dose, and timing are appropriate. Children who do have a delay in weight or height growth see only minor ones, which research has found is made up by the time their growth period is complete

Can stimulant medications cause tics?

This is a rather controversial topic. Tics are involuntary, nonpurposeful, repetitive motor movements or vocalizations. Eye blinking, coughing, snorting, sniffing, and cursing are some examples. Of the 70 to 80 percent of AD/HD children treated with stimulants, it is estimated between 8 and 30 percent develop tics.

Approximately 7 percent of AD/HD children have a coexisting tic disorder. When given stimulant medication, some of these children experience a worsening in tics. In other cases, AD/HD children with no prior existence of tics develop them after they begin to take stimulant medication. Still others develop tics after ceasing the use of stimulant medication.

There is an ongoing debate as to whether or not stimulants unmask tics in AD/HD children who would have developed them anyway, or if the use of stimulants actually causes the tics to start. There is no definitive answer at this point.

Researchers do know, however, that for children whose tics started after using stimulant medication, the tics usually stop for the great majority when the medication is terminated. For this reason, conservative physicians generally stop the use of stimulants and prescribe a different class of medications. Physicians that are more liberal will recommend a second medication to reduce the tics; an option most parents shy away from.

What is sustained released medication?

Sustained or extended release medications involve a once-a-day dose that lasts twelve hours. Instead of the two to four divided doses used for years, sustained release medications have been shown to have a more positive effect for many AD/HD children.

Many parents prefer sustained release medication. These single dose medications eliminate the child's noontime dose at the nurse's office. As these medications provide a steady stream of medication, the child does not experience periods of time when the medication is wearing off and they are waiting for the new pill to take effect. The afternoon rebound that some children experience as their last dose for the day wears off is also eliminated.

Compliance with sustained released medication has been shown to have a rate of 83 percent, a dramatic improvement over the 59 percent compliance rate for divided doses. This translates into parents being more consistent in administering the medication and fewer refusals from their child.

Side effects for sustained release are similar to divided doses. Decreased appetite, stomachaches, insomnia, emotional instability, headaches, and nervousness are the most commonly reported negative effects.

What are the types of nonstimulant medications used?

About one in ten children do not benefit from stimulants. Other classes of medications may be suggested if your child has not responded to stimulants or has been unable to tolerate side effects.

Some physicians will prescribe medication that has been approved only for older children and adults. This is called "off label" use and means that the safety and usefulness of the medication has not been established for the purpose the physician is prescribing. Take time to learn about the medication, its benefits, side effects, and risks.

Straterra is a nonstimulant medication that is frequently prescribed and reported to have a positive benefit for many children. It works on the brain chemical norepinephrine and has generally the same benefits as stimulants.

Tricyclic antidepressants are not a first line of treatment, but may be suggested by your physician if your child is not responsive to stimulants or is unable to tolerate their side effects. Benefits of tricyclics are the absence of potential for abuse and their long acting effect. The downside is the higher risk for side effects.

Antihypertensive drugs are also used in cases of severe hyperactivity, impulsivity, and aggression. Catapress and Tenex are two of the most likely medications in this class.

What are the side effects of nonstimulant medication?

Strattera is reputed to have minimal side effects, some of which are similar to stimulants. Stomachaches, decreased appetite, tiredness, dizziness, and mood swings are the most common side effects. Management of these side effects is similar to stimulant medications. Straterra may show some positive benefits within one to two days, but can take one to three weeks to achieve its full benefit.

Tricyclic antidepressants can result in dry mouth, vivid dreams, headaches, stomachaches, insomnia, and constipation. These medications take one to three weeks before effectiveness is seen. They may not be abruptly stopped and must be decreased under the supervision of a physician. Changes in heart functioning can sometimes occur and thus an EKG (electrocardiogram) may be used in the monitoring process. Blood tests are also part of the monitoring to evaluate blood levels of the medication. Most physicians do not use these medications for prepubescent children. The need for close monitoring of the tricyclics places them low on the list of options for many physicians.

Antihypertensive drugs come in pill or patch form. They may cause fatigue, dizziness, and dry mouth. These medications cannot be abruptly stopped and need to be slowly decreased under the direction of a physician.

Is medication necessary on nonschool days?

For many years, medication for AD/HD was given only on school days. It was believed that children needed a break from the medication. Medication-free weekends, holidays, vacations, and summers gave children a chance to "catch up" on growth in weight and height. Now that delayed growth has been found to be relatively insignificant, the question of taking medication "holidays" is up for debate.

Some physicians encourage parents to give medication to their child only on the days they believe the child needs it. Most often these days are school days, when demands for attention, sustained effort, and decreased physical activity are at their highest.

Other physicians argue that since symptoms do not take a holiday, medication should not take one.

Currently there is no scientific evidence for or against medication holidays. Until researchers have a better understanding of the pros and cons of taking a medication holiday, parents will have to weigh the advantages and disadvantages in cooperation with their prescribing physician. A general guideline followed by some parents is to give medication holidays for children who are relatively free of behavior problems but use the medication primarily for school and homework. Children with severe behavior problems are more likely to remain on medication year-round.

Is the medication addictive?

Stimulant medication does have the potential to be abused when misused. Abusing stimulant medications can lead to addiction. Providing the medication is taken as prescribed, there is not a risk for addiction. Dosages prescribed are low and not anywhere near the amount required to develop a dependency.

There is no tolerance associated with stimulants when used properly—children do not need increasing doses to achieve the same effect. Nonstimulant medications do not have any addictive potential, even if taken in excess. For teens and adults where abuse of medication is a concern, nonstimulant medications offer a safer alternative.

While anyone taking stimulants as prescribed is not going to become addicted to the medication, in one study, one third of teens taking stimulants reported that their non-AD/HD peers had asked them to sell or give them their medication. Over 40 percent of teens surveyed reported that they carried and administered medication to themselves at school, a phenomenon that surely violates every school's policy. While teens do not appear to be abusing their own medication, allowing them to control their own medication may increase the likelihood that they become involved in illegal medication transactions.

Does stimulant medication lead to later drug use?

This is a genuine concern for parents. You are in good company if you have theorized that if your child learns medication is the way to deal with his AD/HD symptoms, he will think medication or drugs are the solution to all his problems. While this theory seems logical, it is not supported by research findings. In fact, just the opposite has been found. Studies have consistently found no association between stimulant medication and increased risk of later drug use in males with AD/HD. Less is known about females.

Long-term studies that followed AD/HD children for a minimum of four years found that stimulant medication reduced the risk for substance abuse by approximately half in adolescents. Teens that remained on medication during adolescence had a lower likelihood of substance use or abuse in their young-adult years.

What are the long-term effects of medication?

Every parent considering medication wonders if his or her child will suffer long-term damage as a result. Stimulants have been used to treat childhood behavior problems since the late 1930s. With the millions of children treated, there are no known permanently damaging effects. To date there have been no known studies suggesting the presence of negative long-term effects.

Unfortunately, the same is true for long-term positive effects. To date there is no research that indicates medication alone alters the child's eventual outcome in adulthood. Medication temporarily alleviates the symptoms; it does not change the child. This lack of positive long-term outcomes for medicated children may be due to medication truly having nothing to offer in the long run. Or it may be a result of research that has typically followed children only a few months to a few years. Longer-term studies in years to come should shed light on whether or not medication simply provides immediate symptom relief or if it alters a child's eventual life outcome.

How long will my child have to take medication?

There are no set timelines to stop medication. This decision will vary for each child. For many years, stimulant medication was only given to children. Adults taking stimulant medication was unheard of until the last decade.

As researchers learn more about medication, it affects the trends in prescribing it. The current trend is to continue medication during adolescence for those teens still showing significant symptoms. Recent research has found teens that remain on medication are substantially less likely to use and abuse drugs and alcohol. Many adults are now taking stimulant medication as they either discover their disorder or become willing to return to medication that helped them as a child.

Many physicians recommend children be given a trial period without medication. Summertime provides a period where consequences of having no medication, if negative, will have less impact than during the school year. Parents and the prescribing physician should have a list of target behaviors to monitor to determine if there is a significant change between medicated and nonmedicated periods. If symptoms are still severe, then a return to medication may be warranted.

How do children feel about taking medication?

Parents are understandably concerned about how their child's self-esteem will be affected by taking medication. The largest concern is that their child will conclude that something is wrong with them.

The limited research that has been done addressing this issue has some very surprising findings. Teens who were taking medication reported that they believed it helped them get along better with their peers. On average, the teens questioned reported that while medication helped their ability to pay attention, they did not believe that the medication helped with their schoolwork. The biggest effect the teens reported was it made their parents like them more. The biggest effect younger children report is that their medication helps them concentrate and/or behave better. They often refer to their medication as a "behavior" pill or "concentration" pill.

Parents concerned that the other students will tease their peers for taking medication can relax. Research indicates that peers don't tend to think negatively of AD/HD students simply because they are taking medication. When they do hold negative views of their AD/HD classmates, it's usually because of repeated, inappropriate classroom and social behavior that the AD/HD child exhibits.

What do I do if my child refuses to take medications?

For most children, taking medication is not a source of conflict. There are some, however, who are resistant and will argue or outright refuse. While their refusal might seem to be just one more defiant behavior, in reality when AD/HD children resist taking medication, there are usually emotional reasons. For many of these children the refusal stems from feeling there is something wrong with them. No child likes to view himself as having "problems," and those with a fragile self-esteem are particularly vulnerable.

Insisting or forcing a child to take his medication may solve the problem in the short run. However, while you win the battle, you lose the war. A private meeting between your child and the prescribing doctor may be all that is needed for her to understand her diagnosis and the benefits of medication. For children who continue to remain resistant, a short course of individual psychotherapy is recommended. Often just a few meetings with a psychologist can uncover and resolve a child's distress about medication.

Does medication teach children that they need pills to succeed?

Studies examining boys' beliefs found they dismiss medication as a contributor to their success. If they succeed on a task, they attribute it to their effort. If they fail, they believe the task was too difficult. Similarly, if boys have positive behavior, they report it being the result of their effort and motivation, not a result of their medication. In fact, boys appear to be overly optimistic that they will have a good day regardless of whether or not they took medication. These findings have mixed consequences. On the one hand, it is positive that the children believe their effort results in their positive behavior. On the other hand, this belief has the potential to result in the children believing that the medication is not helpful and therefore they should not be taking it.

How do parents feel about giving their child medication?

Parents report that deciding to medicate their child was a difficult choice. Feelings of guilt and inadequacy often accompany the decision.

This hesitancy and ambivalence disappear quickly when parents see the noticeable change in their child within thirty minutes of giving them their first dose. The first two weeks of medication often erase any doubts parents previously had. Some parents even feel guilty about not having medicated their child sooner!

This honeymoon phase, however, quickly disappears as the child adjusts to the medication and begins to show his usual symptoms, albeit at a less severe intensity and frequency. Parents experience a great letdown, feeling that the medication has failed them. Their hopes that a pill would solve their child's problems are quickly shattered and the reality of having to really work at parenting sets in.

Research studies show that using medication leads to less satisfaction in the long run for parents who use it as their sole method of treatment. Parents who opt to add medication to a behavioral treatment program report higher and longer-term levels of satisfaction. Those who use combined treatment also remain in treatment longer than those who opt for medication only.

What factors should I consider before giving my child medication?

Medication is an option that must be given careful consideration. Give proper attention to the following issues:

- Has your child had a thorough evaluation?
- Have other disorders been ruled out?
- Have learning disorders been ruled out?
- Have you given behavior modification a serious try?
- Is your child in the proper school setting?
- Have you obtained accommodations and modifications for homework?
- Do you believe in the use of psychiatric medications for children?
- Is your child old enough to safely take medication?

If you have answered "no" to any of the above questions, your child is most likely not suitable for medication at this point in time.

If you answered "yes" to the above questions, consider the following:

- Will medication be one of many treatments you will be using?
- Have you received parent training from an AD/HD specialist?
- Has your child been suspended or expelled?
- Is your child at risk for being expelled?
- Have you lost babysitters due to your child's behavior?
- Is your child violent?

If you have answered "yes" to any of these questions, your child may be a good candidate for medication.

Will I experience pressure to medicate my child?

Medicating your child is one of the most difficult decisions you will face. When you hear "AD/HD," the next word you will hear is "medication." Be prepared to face pressure from other parents, teachers, and doctors.

Teachers may ask, "You wouldn't send him to school without glasses if he needed them, would you? Why would you send him without medication?" Parents may ask you, "Don't you want the best for your child?" Your physician may ask, "You wouldn't deprive your child of insulin would you? Then why would you deprive him of medication?"

Few parents have the fortitude to counter these persuasive arguments. Parents are as guilty as physicians are of using the insulin argument to persuade others who are hesitant to accept medication. The difference between insulin for diabetes and stimulants for AD/HD is that without insulin your child dies. Your child will not die, much less even become sick, without stimulants. A diabetic child has an insulin deficiency. No child has a stimulant medication deficiency. The two disorders and the two medications cannot be compared. They have nothing in common and decisions about medicating your child should not be based on senseless analogies.

How do I resist pressure to give my child medication?

Many adults simply cannot understand why anyone would not jump at the chance to have a pill that improves their child's behavior. When you hear that 70 to 80 percent of children who take medication show improvement, it is hard to resist the temptation to view and use the pill as a solution to your child's behavior problems.

No parent want to medicate his or her child. Many, however, after careful consideration, decide that medication is the right treatment for their child. That does not mean it is the right decision for you and your child.

Parents who decide not to medicate tend to feel more confident in their decision. They are generally more dedicated to behavior management, psychotherapy, and educational interventions. These parents base their decision on the following beliefs:

- Medication is not a cure
- Medication will only decrease some symptoms some of the time
- Medication causes side effects I am not willing to have my child suffer
- Tics may be a side effect I am not willing to risk
- Medication is not a substitute for my effective parenting
- Medication will not make my child learn more
- Medication will not make my child behave

Chapter 8

SOCIAL SKILLS

- Do AD/HD children have poor social skills?
- Do boys' social skills differ from girls'?
- Are social skills different with ADHD in comparison to ADD?
- What are the negative effects of poor social skills?
- How do I recognize if my child has poor social skills?
- How are poor social skills displayed by AD/HD children?
- How does impulsivity affect my child's social skills?
- Can my child learn from negative social experiences?
- Why do AD/HD children have trouble improving social skills?
- How do AD/HD children feel about their social skills?
- Does medication help AD/HD children with their social skills?
- Do children expect medication to help with their social skills?
- How well do AD/HD children read social cues?
- Should I talk to my child about his poor social skills?
- How can I increase positive social skills in my child?
- Should I review social skills with my child?
- Should I make my child accountable for his social behavior?
- How do my social skills influence my child?
- What is social skills therapy?
- Can social skills therapy be helpful?
- What is my role in social skills therapy?
- What do I do when I see my child using poor social skills?
- Should I try to get my child to make more friends?
- How do I help my child make a friend?
- What can schools do to help with social skills?
- How can a buddy program help with social skills?
- Which social skills should I work on with my child?
- Can my child become more likable?

Do AD/HD children have poor social skills?

Social skills are the abilities we use when interacting with others. They are critical to our ability to get along in life. More important than grades, IQ, and academic achievement, the long-term outcome of happiness and success is our ability to determine what is the appropriate behavior in any given situation and the ability to execute the right action.

The majority of children with AD/HD do have poor social skills. Researchers' estimates are that at least 60 percent of children with AD/HD have significant trouble interacting with others. Psychologists working with AD/HD children would put that estimate far higher. Poor social skills are so apparent that children with AD/HD are often rejected by other children after only a single day of contact.

Poor social skills affect both boys and girls with AD/HD. Sadly, AD/HD children of both genders are the most likely to have few friends. In studies examining the friendship patterns of children, those with AD/HD are consistently rated as the least-liked child in their class. When students are given a chance to secretly nominate the one classmate they would not like to play with or invite to their party, the AD/HD child earns the most nominations.

In groups of children who have friends, those with AD/HD are the least likely to have more than one friend. If they are able to make a friend, children with AD/HD have trouble keeping them. Their friendships are unstable and usually short-lived.

Do boys' social skills differ from girls'?

Boys and girls with AD/HD have poor social skills. Because the disorder appears differently in boys than girls, so do the social skills problems.

When boys are observed in activities with a nondisordered male, the boys with AD/HD are more disagreeable, off task, aggressive, and less likely to ask appropriate questions. AD/HD boys who engage in physical aggression against peers have more difficulty making friends, as few are willing to tolerate this behavior. AD/HD boys also tend to be less empathic than non-AD/HD boys. They are less likely to change their behavior to fit the situation. Despite all this, boys tend to overrate their social skills, believing themselves to be more socially adept than is actually the case.

Girls with AD/HD report more social difficulties than boys. They may not actually have more social skills problems, but they appear to be more aware and more distressed by their inability to make and keep friends. Depression is not uncommon in girls who fail to establish at least one friendship. Girls' social deficits show up less in physical activity but more in the interpersonal interaction. Preferring to be the one in charge, AD/HD girls can be bossy and domineering in conversations and play.

Are social skills different with ADHD in comparison to ADD?

ADHD children are much more visible in their social skills deficits than ADD children. Observers can easily pick out those with ADHD in a group of children. Even kindergarten children can identify which children have behavior problems. Studies have shown that some ADHD children are rejected by their peers within moments of meeting. These children are desirous of social interaction and actively seek contact with others. However, the intrusiveness of ADHD children and their failure to read social cues often results in their peers forcefully rejecting them and blatantly insisting they go away.

ADD children are more prone to fade into the background. They tend to be anxious, shy, and withdrawn, which keeps them on the periphery of social activity. Instead of getting into conflict with their peers on the playground, these children are more likely to be alone and play by themselves. When they are interacting with a peer, they can appear "spacey" and "off in their own world." The rejection they experience from their peers is one of quiet avoidance and simply ignoring or forgetting about them. Some ADD children will cope with social rejection by keeping themselves occupied and entertained with reading.

What are the negative effects of poor social skills?

At least half of the children with AD/HD who have social skills problems in childhood continue to have interpersonal problems in adolescence and adulthood, which can lead to a variety of problems. When AD/HD boys with social problems are followed into their adolescence, they are found to have increased mood, anxiety, behavioral, and substance abuse disorders. Even when emotional and behavioral problems are factored out, early social skills problems have been found to be a major contributor to later problems in adolescence.

Early social skills problems in AD/HD children are such a strong predictor of later functioning that even those children who overcome their AD/HD symptoms by adolescence still experience social rejection in their teen years.

Being rejected by peers causes feelings of loneliness, which increases the risk of depression. This also increases the risk for rejected peers to find one another and escalate into antisocial behavior.

Adults with AD/HD rate themselves as less skilled in social skills and relationships. They have trouble reading facial expressions, controlling their verbal responses, and being emotionally overreactive.

How do I recognize if my child has poor social skills?

Parents most often recognize their child's struggle with social skills from listening to their child. As early as kindergarten, some AD/HD children come home from school complaining, "no one likes me," or "nobody will play with me." No parent wants to believe that their child is disliked, so these early complaints often go unheeded.

As other children begin to establish friendships outside of school, the AD/HD child often fails to do so. She does not get invited over to play, birthday party invitations do not come, and no one calls her on the telephone. When she has her own party, she has trouble listing who her friends are and many of those invited find a reason not to come. When she reaches out to her peers, phone calls are not returned and invitations to come over are declined.

Teachers may be the first to identify poor social skills and send home the bad news. The physically aggressive behavior some AD/HD children display on the playground quickly results in their peers not wanting to play with them. Because they can be overactive and intrusive, no one in class seems to want to sit next to them or be their partner on group projects.

How are poor social skills displayed by AD/HD children?

If you were to observe your AD/HD child interacting with a peer, you would probably see several inappropriate social behaviors. He would likely be moving around and paying attention to something other than his peer. When he responds, it will be to interrupt with something unrelated to what his friend was talking about. He may not look at his peer while he talks to him. His talking will not promote a conversation, but rather will be a monologue on his topic of choice. If his peer tries to enter into a dialogue, the AD/HD child will often criticize him and tell him why he is wrong. If they are playing a game, your AD/HD child probably takes charge and bosses the other child. If he begins to lose, he will change the rules. If he loses a turn, he will argue about it and, if his peer does not relent, he will quit playing. He does not want to share or take turns and is insistent that he gets his own way. If things do not go to his liking, he will display his frustration and anger in an outburst with no embarrassment.

How does impulsivity affect my child's social skills?

The very nature of being impulsive means the inability to consistently think before acting. Even if your child does stop to think before he acts, he still must stop himself from doing the wrong thing. Even children with ADD who lack impulsivity as a core symptom tend to have impulsive social behavior.

In social situations, both children with ADD and ADHD fail to think before they say or do something. To get along well with others, we all need to use a mental filter that prompts us to think ahead of time before we say or do something. Children without AD/HD are not much different from those with the disorder. They have inappropriate thoughts and contemplate inappropriate behaviors. The difference is they use their mental filter more consistently and they use an internal voice that guides their decisions. Freud called this internal voice the "superego." It is the voice inside our minds that tell us, "don't throw that rock you could hurt somebody, and you know you will get in trouble. Go ride your bike instead." Children with AD/HD fail to use their internal voice and inhibit their impulses.

Can my child learn from negative social experiences?

AD/HD children can certainly learn from experience. Unfortunately, however, they learn slowly; very, very slowly. What other children may figure out in just one or two situations, AD/HD children can literally take years to learn.

There are several reasons why AD/HD children are slow to profit from their social experiences. One is that they fail to engage in hindsight. Even young children are able to look back at a situation and think about what might have gone wrong. AD/HD children rarely do this spontaneously. When their neighbor does not want to come over to play anymore, they don't stop to contemplate why. They don't look back and try to figure out what went wrong. They have little interest in how yesterday's events effect today.

The second deterrent is their difficulty in linking cause and effect. Even if they are able to use hindsight, they don't link together their behavior and the outcome. The fact that no one wants them to play in the handball game today does not get connected to the fact that yesterday when they missed the ball, they refused to go out of the game.

Why do AD/HD children have trouble improving social skills?

While most children will listen to feedback from parents, teachers, and peers, children with AD/HD outright reject it. It is not uncommon for AD/HD children to spend years rejecting the notion that they have contributed to their social isolation.

All children try to find ways to fit in, trying out different behaviors, roles, and personas. By observing how others react to them, they can determine what results in social acceptance and what results in rejection. AD/HD children, however, fail to observe the reactions of their peers. They try on and continue to engage in a behavior despite it causing rejection by their peers. For example, if they try to fit in by being the class clown, they fail to observe that no one is laughing at their jokes or silly faces.

As AD/HD children grow older, they become more aware of how their peers react to them. They now notice that no one laughs at their goofy faces, but instead of stopping, they simply conclude that no one at their school has a sense of humor. They continue with their attempts at humor, failing to admit that this may be a cause of their social isolation.

How do AD/HD children feel about their social skills?

Despite their poor social skills being quite obvious to everyone else, children with AD/HD are often oblivious to their deficits. When asked to rate their performance on social tasks, children with AD/HD rate themselves as more socially effective than nondisordered children rate themselves. This phenomenon is called a "positive illusory bias."

This positive illusory bias is good news on the one hand; AD/HD children are far more positive about themselves than once believed. On the other hand, their falsely inflated sense of self leaves them blind to their social problems. Everyone around them can easily see why the AD/HD child is rejected, but he has no idea why no one seems to like him. He blames his peers for rejecting him and refuses to accept that his behavior is the problem. The AD/HD child sees nothing wrong in his social behavior and if there is nothing wrong, there is no need for him to do anything differently. While his self-esteem about his own social skills remains high, he is lonely and feels socially isolated. Without recognition and some emotional discomfort, children lack the motivation to change their behavior and improve their social interactions.

Does medication help AD/HD children with their social skills?

This question is up for debate. Many studies have shown that stimulant medication helps to improve the social behavior of children. In particular, aggressiveness and impulsive social behaviors have repeatedly been found to decrease in medicated children.

However, many other studies have failed to find results that extend beyond the decrease in impulsivity and aggressiveness. Medication has been found, in many studies, to have no positive effect on increasing positive social behavior. Nor has it been found to increase skills in good sportsmanship in group games. Most distressing of all to parents is that medication has not been shown to actually increase the number of friends AD/HD children are able to make or keep. The myriad of social problems continues despite the use of medication.

While medication can help to decrease some behaviors, it cannot give your child skills to use in social situations. It is important to keep your expectations of medication realistic. You would not expect an antibiotic to cure an infection, stop appendicitis, and increase the enamel in your child's teeth. Medication helps increase concentration and attention. It does not help your child become more interested in others, more considerate of their feelings, or more willing to accept feedback. Pills do not replace skills.

Do children expect medication to help with their social skills?

Research has found that AD/HD children generally rate their medication as minimal in their social success. Instead, they find their own ability and effort, as well as luck, as the cause of their success or failure. When they fail in a social situation, they are more prone to attribute it to the social task being too difficult, rather than a lack of medication.

Children with AD/HD set their expectations not on the taking or skipping of medication, but whether or not they were recently successful in a social situation. Optimism arises in the shadow of a recent social success, while pessimism is sparked by recent social failure. When researchers study what expectations AD/HD children have about their social success, they find that medication plays no role. Parents tend to place too much emphasis on medication as being the cause of social success or failure, often calling it a "behavior pill."

How well do AD/HD children read social cues?

Social cues are the unspoken behaviors that provide information to guide our responses to others. Facial expressions, eye contact, and tone of voice are examples of social cues. Learning how to read social cues comes naturally to most children simply through experience interacting with others. AD/HD children not only fail to naturally develop these skills, they have great difficulty learning them.

While impulsivity is a major cause of social problems in AD/HD children, their difficulty in reading social cues is likely to be equally responsible. It is not clear if these children fail to read social cues or simply misinterpret them, or a combination of both.

Social cues tend to be subtle and because AD/HD children have trouble recognizing very blatant social feedback, the subtlety of social cues is likely to be easily missed.

AD/HD children also have trouble accurately interpreting facial expressions. They have difficulty identifying how others are feeling and are unable to predict the social behavior of others. They lack the skills necessary to use social cues to guide their own social behavior.

Should I talk to my child about his poor social skills?

Talking to your child is one of the many ways you can help with his social struggles. He will probably give you ample opportunity to discuss his social relationships when he tells you that no one at school likes him. Take care not to give in to your natural parental instincts to rescue your child from his negative feelings. Uncomfortable emotions are often the reason we take a closer look at ourselves and decide to make changes.

Acknowledge his feelings by letting him know that you can see he feels bad. Validate his emotions by telling him that you can understand why he would feel upset. Invite him to explore his experiences by asking him, "Why do you think the children won't play with you?" Encourage him to think about it by prompting more exploratory questions such as, "Is there something you did that you think might have made the other children not want to play with you?"

Do not expect insightful or accurate answers. The goal is to help your child feel comfortable talking about his social conflicts and to instill the need to look at himself to discover the cause and ultimately make changes.

How can I increase positive social skills in my child?

Chances are you have a good idea of which social skills your child struggles with. Make a list of her behavioral excesses and deficits. Don't be surprised if the list is long. Add to it as you observe your child in social situations. AD/HD affects every aspect of social functioning in virtually every setting.

Helping your child increase her social skills is a long-term project. Not every behavior can be addressed at one time. Before your child participates in a social situation, it can be very helpful to review social skills for her to keep in mind. Different situations will call for different skills, giving her plenty of opportunities to work on the various skills. Select two behaviors that you know she struggles with, any more than that can become overwhelming, not to mention easily forgotten. Choose one social skill that is very important for her to do appropriately and a second one that she is likely to perform successfully. Just as you reminded her when she was little how she was to behave in the grocery store, you will have to review for many years how she is to behave in various social settings.

Should I review social skills with my child?

Having discussed and reviewed two social skills before entering a social situation, your child is prepared for a follow up of how things went. Wait until she discusses her experience with you so she doesn't feel like you were watching or grading her. Since we all respond more positively to praise than criticism, your feedback should start with praise.

If she was to work on sharing, you might give her a positive statement such as, "you sure looked like you were having a good time with Jenny. How did the two of you do sharing her toys?" This takes her out of the hot seat and opens up a discussion instead of an interrogation.

If you know she hit her friend, instead of scolding and lecturing her, adopt an exploratory approach that invites her to review in her mind what happened and what she could have done different. Such an invitation might sound like, "I know you hit Jenny when you were playing, what happened?" Listening, acknowledging her viewpoint, and validating her feelings will keep the discussion open, helping her to respond to your query, "What do you think you will do next time you feel so mad at Jenny?"

Should I make my child accountable for his social behavior?

All children should be held accountable for their behavior, including children with AD/HD. Having a disorder does not excuse AD/HD children from taking responsibility for their words and actions. When an AD/HD child has hurt someone, they need to be instructed to try to rectify the relationship. While no child should be purposely humiliated, it is human nature to use our feelings to guide our behavior. The feeling of embarrassment we experience when we have to face the person we hurt is a powerful incentive to alter our behavior in the future. Recalling feelings of shame usually motivates us to restrain our impulses.

Expect your AD/HD child to need repeated experiences of having to "fix the situation." You will not only have to help him see what he did inappropriately and how it made the other person feel, you will have to guide him through the steps of what he needs to do to make it right.

Examples of social behaviors you can prompt and guide your child to be accountable for include:

- Apologizing for teasing
- Saying thank you
- Returning stolen items
- Saying "excuse me" for interrupting
- Apologizing for hitting
- Replacing items broken purposely or accidentally

How do my social skills influence my child?

Poor social skills are an unfortunate side effect of having AD/HD. Parents do not make their child have poor social skills. They can, however, make their child's social skills worse.

Children clearly learn from watching their parents. Parents with hostile and verbally aggressive social styles tend to have children with the same social approach. Parents who are dishonest and manipulative have children who lie and try to get their own way. Parents who are pushy and demanding have children who bully and won't take no for an answer.

What is most interesting to see in clinical practice is how the apple does not fall far from the tree. A parent who brings their child to therapy because they lie, cheat, and throw tantrums to get their own way, usually breaks the twenty-four-hour cancellation rule, lies by saying they left a message, and yells at the receptionist that they won't pay the agreed-upon cancellation fee. They do not put it together that they are doing the very behaviors they want their child to stop.

As a parent of any child, it is important to live the values and behaviors you are trying to instill in your child.

What is social skills therapy?

Social skills therapy is treatment designed to improve social behavior and social relationships. AD/HD children have little ability to identify and discuss the social problems they have, making individual therapy for social skills problems an ineffective treatment. In order to be effective, it must be done in a group setting where the therapist is able to observe your child's interaction with age mates.

Group treatment for social skills has a highly structured format where specific social skills are taught. The children rehearse the skill, role-play in the group, and practice it at home. While the lesson is taking place, the children are interacting with one another, giving the therapist a great opportunity to observe the social strengths and weaknesses of each child.

Appropriate social behaviors are praised in the group to increase the chance of repetition. Inappropriate behaviors are discussed as to the reason, impact, and alternatives. Children are an active part of the group where they give one another feedback about how their behavior appears to others, increasing the chance that the children will select appropriate behavior in order to make friends. Parents must be active participants in the treatment. Homework for parents and children to practice the skills in between sessions is an important component for success.

Can social skills therapy be helpful?

So much emphasis has been placed on the academic functioning of AD/HD children that for decades little attention was paid to their social behavior. Increased understanding that AD/HD children have poor social skills has lead to the development of treatment programs designed to improve social functioning.

Findings have been mixed, with some studies showing improvement and others finding little to none. This does not mean social skills treatment is ineffective, but is likely to be more a reflection of the fact that studies have focused largely on short-term success—usually just several months.

How researchers define social success also determines whether treatment is helpful. When popularity is used as the definition of success, treatment clearly does not work. However, if researchers look at the actual increase in the number and frequency of appropriate social behaviors, success can be expected.

As any clinician will tell you, changing social skills is a long-term project. AD/HD children are very weak in their social skills and very slow to make changes. More success is likely to be seen when the social functioning is measured years and decades down the road and the number of skills, effectiveness, and frequency of skills is the definition of success.

What is my role in social skills therapy?

Social skills therapy focuses on teaching and rehearsing various social behaviors in a group setting. This alone has only moderate impact. You must be involved in the treatment in order for the lessons to become integrated into your child's repertoire of behavior. You must be active in prompting your child to practice the skills.

Effective treatment programs include educating parents about the skills their child is learning. Through written handouts for parents and homework for children, specific social skills are to be practiced outside the treatment setting. The more enthusiasm parents show about using the social skills, the more eager the children are. The more the parents use the skills themselves, the more likely it is that their child will also use them.

When parents are assigned by the group leader to make play dates with another child in the group, those parents who take an active role in making and monitoring the play dates have children who report higher satisfaction with their new friend than children whose parents have little involvement. The more parents work to arrange play dates, the higher the quality of the friendships the children are able to establish.

What do I do when I see my child using poor social skills?

The more you supervise your child's social interactions, the greater chance you have to help her become aware of her errors and correct them. So that your child does not feel embarrassed by your calling attention to her social errors, you and she can develop a secret signal to use when you observe her behaving in a socially inappropriate manner.

Your child may respond well to a subtle visual signal such as you tugging on your earlobe or scratching your nose. Physical touch can also cue your child to stop and think about his behavior. Agree on a specific touch that you only use when cueing him to change what he is doing. Three taps on the shoulder or a gentle rub on the back of his neck. Verbal code words can also be used. For children who need repeated reminders to use appropriate social skills, it is more effective to choose one code word you can whisper in her ear.

Be sure to ask your child what signal he would like you to use. If your child chooses the signal, he is more likely to watch for it and respond.

Should I try to get my child to make more friends?

Given that social skills deficits are a rather serious problem for children with AD/HD, the likelihood of them being able to make more friends is small. The situation for many AD/HD children is that they do not have even one consistent friend. Psychologists thus believe that rather than trying to increase the number of friends or increase overall popularity, a more realistic goal is to try to help your child develop one solid friendship.

Children who develop just one friendship are happier than those who have none. Having a friend at school to be with at recess and lunchtime provides pleasure, prevents loneliness, and decreases the frequency of being targeted for teasing and bullying.

For children who are unable to develop a friendship at school, parents should provide opportunities to meet other children who may turn into a friend. Knowing she has a friend to play with after school, spend the night with on the weekend, or call on the telephone can make the loneliness at school easier to tolerate and give her something to look forward to.

Neighbors, cousins, teammates, church members, and children involved in your child's outside activities are potential friends.

How do I help my child make a friend?

Focusing on quality not quantity, parents can be helpful in their child's social life. Your child may be too uncomfortable to call a friend on the phone or ask them in person to get together. Rather than push him into this behavior, arrange with the other child's parent for a get-together. Let your child work on simply getting along well enough that the other child will want to play together again.

Invite various children over until your child finds someone who he gets along well with. Social skills group therapy is a good place to work on finding a friend, as the other children and parents are looking for friends too.

Because many children with AD/HD have extremely delayed skills in cooperative play and anger management, their play dates need to take this into account and plan for it. Structure the activities and your expectations according to your child's social and emotional abilities, not his age. If he is prone to yell, hit, argue, and throw tantrums like a preschool child, choose an activity that decreases the opportunities for these behaviors.

What can schools do to help with social skills?

The two most painful school memories reported by adults are the loneliness they felt while wandering the campus alone at lunch-time and the teasing and taunting they endured from their peers. To prevent today's AD/HD children from years of daily emotional hurt, the creation of a "lunch club" is the easy, no-cost answer.

A lunch club is simply a room for children to go to under the supervision of a teacher or parent volunteer. In the lunch club, the children eat their lunch together and play games or work on a project or activity that they select. At a minimum, loneliness is eliminated and at a maximum, friendships may develop, happiness is increased, and confidence is raised.

Teachers can help AD/HD children be seen in a more positive light by highlighting their talents. Providing the AD/HD child an opportunity to shine in front of his peers can help create common interests that may foster the development of a friendship.

Your child's social value can also be increased by having him perform a simple task. Handing out stickers to each child who turned in their homework can provide him the opportunity for his peers to associate him with a positive experience. You can work with the teacher to create positive social experience opportunities for your child.

How can a buddy program help with social skills?

Children who are rejected by their peers eventually become despondent and give up trying to make friends. They opt to eat lunch alone and aimlessly wander the playground while their peers have fun playing with one another. Schools can prevent continued peer rejection by creating a buddy program.

Buddy programs can include students in leadership and/or any student who is interested in volunteering. Buddies meet under teacher or parent volunteer supervision and identify which students are bullied, rejected, and teased. Each "buddy" selects one of the students to make friends with. The buddy tells his own group of peers that he will be inviting the student to join the social circle and enlists their support. The buddy invites their student to eat lunch with him and join his group in after-lunch play or socializing.

Students who have participated in a buddy program have been found to have a sense of social belonging. With the increased sense of self-worth that comes from being accepted by peers, the students have new-found motivation to improve other aspects of their lives, such as grades and behavior. Students invited by the buddy often then extend their own invitation to a peer they see who is lonely and rejected.

Which social skills should I work on with my child?

Many of the social skills that AD/HD children are deficient in are skills that come easier to other children. While all children need to be taught, prompted, and praised for using proper social behavior, AD/HD children require several years of reminders to use basic social skills.

You can prompt your child to engage in the following behaviors:

- Looking people in the eye
- Waiting his turn to talk
- Greeting others hello
- Staying on topic in conversations
- Saying thank you with meaning
- Acknowledging and accepting compliments
- Not touching others to get their attention
- Taking turns in play
- Saying goodbye when departing
- Sitting still while talking with others
- Responding relevantly to what others have said
- Showing an interest in others by asking questions
- Giving compliments
- Asking peers to join them in play
- Sharing toys, games, and food
- Letting others talk
- Smiling when greeting others
- Listening to others
- Letting others go first
- Apologizing when appropriate
- Showing empathy

Can my child become more likable?

Fortunately, there are many ways to be likeable. If your child can develop character traits that are highly valued by others, it can help make up for some of her more unpleasant social behaviors. Talking about the importance of character can emphasize to your child aspects of himself that she may be able to develop; aspects that she may find easier than controlling her symptoms of AD/HD. Her grades in fourth grade will not have a life-long impact on her, but the development of her character will.

Take every opportunity you find to point out your admiration of these traits in your child and in others. Even movie characters present opportunities to discuss character traits. The good news about character development is that it is under your child's control. He may not be able to stop himself from interrupting others, but he can control how honest he is and how loyal he remains to his friends.

People of high character are likeable. The following characteristics are those found in highly likeable people:

- Loyal
- Truthful
- Dependable
- Thoughtful
- Reliable
- Warm
- Understanding
- Honest
- Humorous
- Sincere
- Cheerful
- Happy
- Unselfish
- Trustworthy
- Responsible
- Friendly

Chapter 9

SELF-ESTEEM

- Does AD/HD affect self-esteem?
- How much self-esteem do AD/HD children have?
- How do I tell if my child has low self-esteem?
- Do all children with AD/HD have low self-esteem?
- Can a child have too much self-esteem?
- Can inflated self-esteem be helpful?
- What is the long-term outlook of self-esteem for AD/HD children
- How will special education affect my child's self-esteem?
- How can my child's teacher help with self-esteem?
- How does teasing affect self-esteem?
- How can I help my child cope with being teased?
- Can extracurricular activities increase self-esteem?
- Can praise increase self-esteem?
- How can compliments increase self-esteem?
- How does my parenting style affect my child's self-esteem?
- How can unconditional love help with self-esteem?
- Can material goods increase self-esteem?
- Can helping others increase my child's self-esteem?
- How can I help my child stop negative self-talk?
- How can I help my child accept his weaknesses?
- How do I give my child a realistic sense of self?
- How do I help my child find a sense of competence?
- How can "snapshots" increase my child's self-esteem?
- What factors are associated with high self-esteem?

Does AD/HD affect self-esteem?

Having any type of psychological disorder can have a negative effect on self-esteem. AD/HD in particular is far more vulnerable than other disorders. Most other disorders in children are not so easily seen by people. As long as others do not know he has a disorder, the child can avoid embarrassment. AD/HD, on the other hand, cannot be hidden. The overt behaviors displayed by the AD/HD child are frequently responded to with negative comments by others. Both the inability to hide the disorder and the negative feedback he receives contributes to feelings of low self-worth.

Further contributing to negative self-esteem is that, unlike other disorders, AD/HD does not elicit sympathy. While a depressed child might be treated with more kindness and patience, the AD/HD engenders frustration and impatience. Being told repeatedly to "stop moving," "stop interrupting," or "stop talking so much" leads the AD/HD child to feel as if he is always doing something wrong. This, of course, leads to lower self-esteem.

Esteem issues are problematic for both ADD and ADHD children. Neither disorder appears to have a better outcome than the other.

How much self-esteem do AD/HD children have?

Self-esteem is not a black and white situation of having or not having it. Nor is it something that can really be measured as to how much a child has. Rather, it is on a continuum from low to high. Unfortunately, having AD/HD often places the child closer to the low end in their overall feelings of self-worth. AD/HD children often have low self-esteem in the main categories of school, family, and friends.

The good news is that these are not the only areas where children can find positive feelings of self-worth. Fortunately, children do not have just one self-esteem. As early as preschool, children are able to make assessments about how they feel about themselves in a variety of areas. The level of overall self-esteem can be increased by adding to the number of arenas your child has a chance to find success in.

You can help your child develop multiple self-esteems. The more activities and experiences he has in which he feels good about himself, the higher his overall level of self-esteem is going to be. As many AD/HD children shy away from new experiences, particularly those that involve the potential for failure or social rejection, be sure to create simple experiences that offer a high chance of success.

How do I tell if my child has low self-esteem?

Children with low self-esteem will reveal their level of self-esteem through their words. Listen to what your child says about himself. Children with low self-esteem talk negatively about themselves and to themselves. Examples of such statements include:

- I'm stupid
- Everybody hates me
- I'm not good at anything
- Nobody cares if I am alive
- I'm ugly

Your child will also reveal her level of self-esteem through her behavior. Watch how she reacts to compliments, criticism, and defeat. Children with low self-esteem are uncomfortable with compliments. They do not believe the compliment is true and therefore are unwilling to accept it with a thank you. Instead, they tend to break eye contact and shy away, either saying nothing or rejecting the compliment by berating themselves.

When criticized, children with low self-esteem have difficulty accepting the negative feedback. Because their self-esteem is so fragile, the slightest indication that they have a fault stimulates a global sense of failure to which they react with anger. Handling difficult tasks and failure also is very distressing for AD/HD children with low self-esteem. Their frustration tolerance is very low and their temper flares rapidly if they are not immediately successful.

Do all children with AD/HD have low self-esteem?

Despite all the concern about low self-esteem, there is research that shows that many boys with AD/HD actually have over-inflated self-esteem. Less is known about the self-esteem of girls with AD/HD.

When asked to rate their scholastic competence, social acceptance, and behavior, many boys with AD/HD overestimate themselves in all areas. In fact, a large number of AD/HD boys who have notable aggression problems or low academic achievement overestimate their competence even more than AD/HD boys without aggression. Their inflated self-esteem follows a pattern of rating themselves highest in areas where they actually function the weakest. ADHD boys with the lowest academic achievement tend to give themselves the highest academic competence ratings.

Almost all very young children overestimate their abilities. As they grow, they begin to develop more accurate self-appraisals. AD/HD children, however, may not alter their over-inflated sense of self as they get older. Some continue to overestimate their own abilities, perhaps in a self-protective manner to compensate for their true feelings of incompetence. The more hyperactive and impulsive the child, the more they tend to overestimate their competence. It thus seems that for many boys, having AD/HD results in more of a falsely inflated sense of self than low self-esteem.

Can a child have too much self-esteem?

Thinking too highly of yourself turns out not to be such a good thing. When people think too highly of themselves, we may label them as conceited, narcissistic, or egotistical. Just as adults can believe themselves to be more worthy than others view them, so too can children. These children tend to be disliked by others, viewed as a "know it all," condescending, and critical of others. AD/HD children often fall into these categories.

Too much self-esteem prevents the AD/HD child from being able to learn from feedback from others. While a child with healthy self-esteem may feel a bit hurt when no one on the playground is interested in talking to him about his dinosaur collection, the AD/HD child determines that no one in class is smart enough to know anything about dinosaurs. He regards himself as highly intelligent and an expert in dinosaurs and derives positive self-esteem from this self-perception. He does not bother to consider that the reason no one is talking to him about dinosaurs is because that is all he ever talks about. He does not piece together that his talk about dinosaurs is boring and actually makes his peers avoid him and maybe he should find a more common topic to talk about. Instead, he holds tightly to his distorted and falsely inflated self-esteem and therefore fails to make any changes in his behavior.

Can inflated self-esteem be helpful?

The lack of awareness of one's own deficits characterizes AD/HD children. They have a remarkable inability to accurately observe themselves. We do not know if this inability is simply the result of being unaware of themselves, or if it is a purposeful defense against the emotional pain that comes from admitting their weaknesses. Or perhaps they overrate themselves because they simply do not know the difference between successful and unsuccessful performance.

While we do not know the exact process, we do know that many children with AD/HD suffer from excessive, rather than low, self-esteem. These children may not be lying about their abilities, but instead deceiving themselves in order to avoid feelings of inadequacy.

This can be a protective mechanism that helps the AD/HD child to preserve his sense of adequacy. If he were to internalize all the negative feedback he hears each day, he would not have the emotional fortitude to even get out of bed.

If your child exaggerates his abilities and worthiness, it is best to not burst his bubble, as he would not be doing this if he did not need the positive feelings it brings. Your best efforts are in encouraging his strengths and helping him accept his weaknesses.

What is the long-term outlook of self-esteem for AD/HD children?

Adults with AD/HD are less likely to express a positive self-image. Greater than two thirds of surveyed adults without AD/HD report having a bright outlook on their future, in comparison to less than half of adults who have AD/HD. More than 75 percent of adults without AD/HD report that they like being themselves and accept themselves for who they are. In dramatic contrast, only half of adults with AD/HD report the same self-perceptions.

While the exact cause for the continued low self-esteem in adulthood is not clear, the general life functioning of adults who continue to have AD/HD is rather poor. They have more divorces, more frequent job changes, less educational achievement, more arrests, more drug and alcohol abuse, and more stress and depression than their non-AD/HD counterparts. These negative life experiences certainly contribute to lower self-esteem. Low self-esteem in turn creates a risk for these negative life experiences to occur.

Children and teens that grow out of the disorder have self-esteem on par with their nondisordered peers. Even those who maintain the disorder have a high chance for good self-esteem if they learn to manage their symptoms and learn compensatory skills and coping tools.

How will special education affect my child's self-esteem?

One of the first questions parents have when special education is recommended is, "How will it affect my child's self-esteem?" Opinions are mixed as to whether or not special education has a positive, negative, or neutral effect on children's self-esteem.

How your child's self-esteem is affected by special education will vary depending on the unique aspects of your child, her educational needs, and the individual aspects of the special education setting.

If special education has been recommended, you need to evaluate how your child is coping emotionally, socially, and behaviorally in the mainstream classroom. If your child is frequently in trouble in the classroom, unable to follow rules, and rejected by her peers, chances are she has low self-esteem. If she remains in the same environment, she has little opportunity to change the way she feels about herself. However, if she moves to a special education classroom that is structured for her to stay out of trouble and places her with similar peers with whom she can make friends, her self-esteem is likely to increase.

How can my child's teacher help with self-esteem?

A good portion of a negative sense of self has its roots on the school campus. Children with AD/HD have difficulty getting through the school day without receiving negative feedback. Reprimands in the classroom and teasing on the playground both contribute to low self-esteem.

Teachers can be of great help in your child's self-esteem with praise and encouragement. Ideas for your child's teacher can include:

- Creating a no-teasing rule in the class and on the playground
- Publicly praising your child to enhance him in the view of his classmates
- Ensuring that teasers apologize to your child
- Giving praise for effort
- Assigning your child a special job to help her feel important
- Reading stories to the class that teach empathy and promote kindness
- Creating a "you're a star" program for students to write compliments on a paper star and hang on the classroom bulletin board
- Giving a weekly "friendship award" to one student who exhibits true friendship
- Appointing your child as the classroom expert on a topic he excels in
- Looking for ways to praise frequently
- Creating a compliment program for students to publicly praise one another in class

How does teasing affect self-esteem?

"Sticks and stones may break my bones, but words can never hurt me," is a familiar phrase every child learns early on to protect their self-esteem against the sting of teasing.

Every child is teased at some point in his or her childhood. AD/HD children often are the brunt of more than their fair share of name-calling and ridicule.

Unfortunately, AD/HD children are also the most ill-equipped to cope with being teased. Their lack of impulse control, aggressiveness, limited frustration tolerance, and poor social skills increase the risk of inappropriate responses. The immature responses that AD/HD children give when teased cause even more problems, often leading to more teasing, increased rejection, and consequences from parents and teachers.

For many adults who have low self-esteem, they flag the teasing they endured in school as a major cause of their suffering years later. Being called names, teased, bullied, and rejected hurts in the immediate moment and can hurt for days, months, and years later. It is thus critical that children with AD/HD learn how to respond to teasing in the presence of their peers and learn how to cope with it internally so that it does not destroy their self-esteem.

How can I help my child cope with being teased?

One of children's biggest complaints about being teased is that adults do not do anything to help. Children are told to work it out themselves; yet, they do not possess the knowledge, skills, and impulse control to work it out.

They are also told to just ignore it. Any frequently teased child will tell you that ignoring simply does not work. Children who tease others can be relentless and have far more stamina in their teasing than your AD/HD child has in ignoring it.

Help your child understand that the reason he keeps getting teased is because he reacts. His reaction is like a jackpot on a slot machine, urging the teaser to keep going. Encourage your child not to be a reactor, but instead to be a joiner. Joining in the teasing with laughter and agreement can stop the payoff the teaser is seeking.

Your child can disarm the teaser with some humorous phrases of agreement. Some examples include:

- Thank you for noticing!
- I know, I wish I could be more like you!
- You got that right!
- I can't argue with that!
- What can I say?
- Don't I know it!
- You are so right!

Can extracurricular activities increase my child's self-esteem?

School for many AD/HD children represents an arena of failure and rejection that they cannot escape. Activities outside of school can provide an environment to preserve and enhance self-esteem.

Self-esteem found in other arenas can make up for the despondency many AD/HD children feel at school. Success at an activity other than school can provide feelings of accomplishment, pride, and motivation. Outside activities can also provide an opportunity for your child to have positive interactions with other children.

Any outside activity that your child enjoys can increase self-esteem. It is the pleasure of the activity, not their ability, that generates self-esteem. Sports have been repeatedly shown to enhance self-esteem. Participants in athletic activities have better images of their own bodies, higher levels of self-esteem, and more trust in others. Girls in particular learn to appreciate their bodies and the fact that strength and endurance are assets. Participation in sports teaches children not just how to win, but how to lose. Sports teach children how to work with others and set goals. Not every AD/HD child is able to function in team sports due to their symptoms. Individual sports like golf, gymnastics, track, and horseback riding provide benefits without the stress of intense social interaction.

Can praise increase self-esteem?

Indiscriminate praise is meaningless. Praise is only meaningful when it is based on your child's actual effort and performance. When children are praised regardless of how hard they tried or how much success they achieved, the praise becomes empty.

The purpose of praise is to engender positive feelings about oneself. The hope is that those positive feelings become part of your child's identity. When he is flattered about everything, he has no way to form a realistic sense of self. He knows he is not good at every-thing and knows he does not put forth equal effort in everything he tries. Yet, if he is being positively reinforced for everything he does, he comes to disbelieve the praise, even when it is well deserved.

Praise is important and feels good, but what really matters is how your child praises himself. He learns from your realistic feedback how to talk to himself about his good points and weak points, as well as his efforts. Your praise is most effective when it is truthful. Your child will mimic your praise when he is assessing himself in his mind. He will have a positive and accurate self-appraisal if you have helped him learn to evaluate his effort and performance in a realistic manner.

How can compliments increase self-esteem?

Compliments make most people feel good about themselves. AD/HD children are hungry for compliments, but are often the least likely to receive them. The goal of compliments is to help your child feel competent and increase the chance he will repeat the behavior.

Compliments need to be truthful and genuine. False compliments can easily be detected by children—particularly those given by their parents. Compliment only when your child earned it with his effort or performance.

Since compliments belong to the receiver, they need to be about the receiver. Rather than telling your child how proud you are of him, tell him you hope he is proud of himself. You want him to be able to feel his own pride so that he will want to repeat the behavior and take pride in himself.

Make compliments only about praise, not an opportunity to teach, coach, or motivate. "You did a great job cleaning your room!" is only a compliment if you don't add, "why can't you do it like this every time?" Compliment and stop talking.

How does my parenting style affect my child's self-esteem?

Authoritarian parents enforce rules but often at the expense of their child's emotions. They use force and punishment to control their child, withdrawing and rejecting them when they disobey. These children tend to be anxious, withdrawn, and unhappy. Their social interactions are hostile and they are easily angered and defiant.

Permissive parents are nurturing, but at the expense of imposing control on their child. They allow their child to make decisions regardless of the child's ability to do so. They have little structure and are permitted to behave as they choose. These children tend to be behaviorally out of control, incapable of controlling their impulses, disobedient, and rebellious.

In contrast, parents who use an authoritative style have children that are happy, self-confident, and self-controlled. Authoritative parenting involves parents who make reasonable demands for behavior enforced by setting limits and insisting on obedience. Failure to obey consistently results in appropriate consequences. When their children are defiant, authoritative parents are patient and rational. They do not give in or respond harshly, but use reasonable, firm control with warmth and affection. Children raised by authoritative parents usually become adolescents who retain high self-esteem, academic success, social maturity, and high moral achievement.

How can unconditional love help with self-esteem?

Almost every person is desirous of acceptance by others. Those who are rejected become even needier. Imagine having no one in your life who accepts you the way you are. Each encounter you have in your life leaves you with the feeling that you are different, you cause problems, and you frustrate others, causing them to not want to be around you.

It is immeasurably helpful for your child to have a safe haven to come home to. Knowing when he gets home he will be accepted and loved can help him get through a tough day at school. A home where he knows he is accepted for who he is with all his symptoms and quirks provides a safe harbor from the harshness of life outside the home.

If your child has significant symptoms, you can be sure he is not getting unconditional acceptance outside the home; so you must be sure to give it in the home. If you do not give him unconditional love, then who will?

If you accept him and he feels this, he will come to accept and love himself and search for this in his friends. He learns he is worthy, despite his symptoms.

Can material goods increase self-esteem?

Material goods surely can bring us pleasure, but they do not make us a person of good character and high esteem. AD/HD children are more prone to fall into the trap of materialism. More than the nondisordered child, AD/HD children use their belongings to attempt to attract and keep friends. They may give away their items, use toys to entice peers to play with them, or threaten to take away a shared item if their peer plays with another child.

How one finds their self-esteem will ultimately determine how happy they are with themselves. Our current culture places quite an emphasis on pursuing happiness and enhanced self-esteem through money and material goods. Any parent who has succumbed to their child's pressure to buy the latest athletic shoe worn by their favorite sports star will tell you that the happiness was short-lived. Your child is happy for a few days in his new shoes. He feels good when his peers marvel at his new shoes, but inside those shoes, he is still the same person. He either learns to like who he is or he just gets hungry for something else to feed his appetite to feel good about himself.

Can helping others increase my child's self-esteem?

It is human nature to want to help others. Helping another person can engender great feelings of competence, pride, self-worth, and satisfaction, feelings your child likely does not find at school.

There are many places where your child can volunteer to help others. Many schools have created programs for AD/HD students to help. Since many AD/HD children get along much better with younger children, schools have harnessed this skill and provided mid and late elementary school students opportunities to be a teacher's helper in kindergarten and first grade classrooms. Reading to the class, tutoring, or playing games with the younger students can give the AD/HD child a sense of competence. He will also be in an environment where he is liked, admired, and the children are excited to see him.

Even though AD/HD children might be rejected by their peers, they are often adored by adults. Your child can receive positive feedback from visiting retirement and nursing homes. He can read to the residents, bring a therapy dog, entertain them with a talent, or play board games. He will learn about kindness to others while receiving positive feedback from grateful seniors who are otherwise without the joy that a child brings.

How can I help my child stop negative self-talk?

We all have an internal voice we use to talk to ourselves. This "self-talk" is how we give ourselves feedback. We each have statements we are prone to repeat to ourselves over and over, as if we made a tape recording and repeatedly press play.

Children with high self-esteem have positive self-talk. Those with low self-esteem and/or depression engage in more negative self-talk.

You are likely to hear your child criticize himself. When you hear your child say something such as, "I'm stupid," instead of telling him that he is wrong, a more helpful approach is to help him talk about why he feels this way. Once he explains the situation that is causing him to feel stupid, you will be able to offer a more reality-based counter statement. You may respond with, "sounds more like you feel you are bad at doing fractions, not that you are stupid." This helps put his negative self-talk in a more realistic perspective. He may indeed be poor at doing fractions, something he will have to work on, but he is not altogether stupid. Eventually he will learn to have this talk within himself.

How can I help my child accept his weaknesses?

Parents sometimes make the mistake of trying to make their child feel they are good at everything. This false feedback will result in your child having a distorted sense of self. Children need to learn to appraise themselves accurately.

When your child expresses negative self-talk that is accurate, it can be helpful to assist them in accepting the negative aspect of themselves. If your child is truly poor at soccer, there are several responses that may be of help: "Would you like to be better at soccer?" showing him that the situation might be temporary. "Is it important to you to be good at soccer?" prompts him to realize he does not have to be good at everything. Asking, "Is there something you feel that you are really good at?" helps him change the focus from the negative to the positive. Offering these concepts in question form is better than simply telling him that he does not have to be good at everything, or that he shouldn't worry because he is good at horseback riding. Questions teach him the process of evaluating himself and his negative self-talk so that eventually he can do it on his own.

How do I give my child a realistic sense of self?

As a parent, you have a dramatic effect on your child's self-esteem. Your encouragement when he is discouraged provides a temporary voice that tells him to keep going until he is able to tell that to himself. Every child must master the emotions of defeat, being able to persevere when things get tough and keep coming back despite failure. Children with a realistic sense of self do not become shattered when they do not succeed and are able to use self-talk to soothe their upset feelings.

Your child will develop a realistic sense of self from mirroring what you tell him. Honest feedback is what works. Praise in times of success is easy. It is in times of defeat that it is most difficult to help your child maintain his self-esteem. Some reality-based encouraging words might include, "I know you are disappointed, but..."

- You sure looked like you were really trying hard
- You put forth a really good effort and that's what really counts
- It's the fun of it that is important, not the outcome
- You can be proud of yourself for hanging in there
- You are handling your upset really well

How do I help my child find a sense of competence?

We all need to feel that we are competent at something. The more things your child feels good about doing, the more feelings of competence she will have, leading to increased self-esteem.

Find opportunities to point out to your child the things she is good at. She does not have to earn the first place ribbon to be good at her sport. She can be good at consistently showing up to the game, praising her teammates, showing enthusiasm for the game, or keeping her chin up when the team loses.

Look for all the ways she is good, not just the obvious. Your verbal recognition will eventually be replaced by her self-acknowledgement.

Your child can also be competent in character traits. She need not have a talent or skill to experience competence. She can feel competence in her friendship skills if she is honest, loyal, and stands up for her friends when they are teased. She can experience feelings of competence as a charitable person when she donates her toys to a children's charity.

How can "snapshots" enhance my child's self-esteem?

"Snapshots" are moments when your child shines above his usual functioning. They are moments of increased feelings of competence. Starting with show-and-tell in kindergarten, teachers use snapshots to create opportunities for each child to stand out in a positive light. School plays, track meets, award ceremonies, and certificates of accomplishment are familiar snapshots schools create to showcase their students and provide opportunities for feelings of enhanced esteem.

AD/HD children need numerous snapshots to sustain their feelings of self-worth in between the big events. Work with your child's teacher to find ways for your child to experience additional snapshots. Create opportunities for your child to display a particular talent or interest in his class and perhaps other classrooms. Mentioning your child's unique talent, interest, or experience in the school newspaper gives public recognition, good feelings for your child, and a trinket for his scrapbook of accomplishments.

What factors are associated with high self-esteem?

People with high self-esteem have a variety of abilities that allow them to remain feeling positive about themselves regardless of the challenges they face, the failure they may experience, or the criticism they receive. Abilities you can foster in your child to work toward increasing self-esteem include:

- Willingness to try new experiences
- Using positive self-talk
- Confidence to try
- Ability to accept compliments
- Comfort with the reality that they cannot be good at everything
- Perseverance when things get tough
- Belief in themselves that if they keep trying, they have a chance at success
- Feeling comfortable saying "I'm not good at…"
- Focusing on what they are good at instead of what they are not
- Separating areas of weakness from overall worthiness
- Understanding criticism does not mean he is a failure
- Not fearing failure
- Measure success based on effort, fun, and experience rather than the outcome
- Having multiple self-esteems

Chapter 10

GROWING UP WITH AD/HD

- How does AD/HD change over time?
- How many children outgrow AD/HD by adolescence?
- How many adolescents outgrow AD/HD by adulthood?
- How far in school are AD/HD children likely to go?
- What does the employment future look like for AD/HD children?
- What types of careers are AD/HD children likely to succeed in?
- What is the risk for AD/HD children to smoke?
- What is the risk for AD/HD children to use alcohol?
- What is the risk for AD/HD children to use drugs?
- What factors increase the risk of drug use in AD/HD teens?
- What is the risk for drug use in adults with AD/HD?
- Are there factors that reduce the risk of drug use?
- What is the risk of acting out behavior for AD/HD teens?
- What is the sexual behavior of AD/HD teens and adults?
- What are the chances for AD/HD teens and adults to engage in crime?
- What is the risk of auto accidents for AD/HD teens and adults?
- What is the likelihood of AD/HD teens developing Antisocial Personality Disorder?
- What are the chances of my child having a successful marriage?
- What kind of parents do AD/HD adults make?
- What is the risk for AD/HD children to develop emotional problems as an adult?
- What can parents do to ensure a good future for their child?
- Can AD/HD be a strength?
- What is the good news about AD/HD?
- Can AD/HD be a gift?

How does AD/HD change over time?

We now know that AD/HD spans throughout childhood and adolescence and often into adulthood. As each person with AD/HD grows older and naturally matures, symptoms change despite the continued presence of the disorder.

Symptoms of ADHD start out highly visible and over time become less noticeable to the outside observer. Preschool and early elementary children with ADHD are usually identified because they appear to have a relentless supply of energy that prompts them to be highly physically active regardless of the circumstances. As they enter into the middle years of elementary school, their symptoms typically manifest less in excessive gross motor movements but more in fidgeting, inattentiveness, and impulsivity. School remains a challenge for most ADHD children and teens.

ADD starts out invisible to the outside observer and stays invisible. Daydreaming, distractibility, forgetfulness, and the inability to complete tasks looks like laziness in children and teens. In adults, ADD looks like a disorganized, scattered, and easily bored person who cannot be counted on to follow through on things.

Those who learn how to function with their symptoms have a better adjustment. Those who fail to develop an awareness of their symptoms and learn coping tools are at high risk for a negative outcome.

How many children outgrow AD/HD by adolescence?

When AD/HD was first defined as a diagnosis under various different names, such as hyperkinesis or minimal brain dysfunction, it was thought that most children outgrew the disorder in their early teens. If a teenager retained a few symptoms after puberty, they were thought to disappear by the end of their teen years. The focus in the earlier years was on hyperactivity, thus as teens matured and were no longer excessively hyperactive, they were thought to have outgrown the disorder.

As research progressed and children were followed into adolescence, the belief that the majority of children outgrew the disorder by puberty was discarded. The new belief was that one third out grew the disorder by adolescence, another third by adulthood, and only one third retained significant symptoms into adulthood.

Ongoing studies in recent years have extended the length of time researchers follow children with AD/HD. As these children grow into adolescence, many of them continue to have the disorder. Current estimates indicate that AD/HD continues to be present in 65 to 70 percent of adolescents who were diagnosed in childhood. As a result, treatment is now recommended to continue throughout adolescence.

How many adolescents outgrow AD/HD by adulthood?

Unfortunately, we are far away from knowing how many adults continue to retain the disorder. Estimates are so wide in range as to be meaningless, with some studies showing as little as 10 percent and other studies showing as many as 70 percent.

One cause for the difficulty is that it depends on who is reporting. When adults who were known to have AD/HD in childhood were asked if they still had the disorder, only 5 percent stated yes. When the parents of these same adults were asked if their child still had AD/HD in their adult years, the response is remarkably different, with 58 percent of parents indicating that their adult child still has the disorder.

Another difficulty in obtaining an accurate estimate is the fact that the symptoms are all normal behaviors that most adults engage in at various times. Every adult from time to time feels distracted, is forgetful, impatient, and bored by tedious tasks. It is normal to daydream, lose a belonging, and feel restless. If we simply went down the checklist, almost every adult on the planet would have AD/HD. The adult symptoms must cause impairment in functioning in order to be diagnosed with AD/HD.

How far in school are AD/HD children likely to go?

The many academic challenges AD/HD children have increase their risk for dropping out of high school. The boredom, tediousness of homework, and the lack of excitement in learning becomes too much for some disordered teens. Paired with poor social relationships and low peer acceptance, some AD/HD teens fail to find school a rewarding place to be. Children with AD/HD are far more likely to fail to graduate from high school. The national average for high school dropouts is approximately 9 percent. The rate is twice that for those with AD/HD. High school dropouts are three times more likely than graduates to earn a poverty income.

With ever increasing numbers of adolescents thought to retain many of their symptoms, more college students are found to have AD/HD than previously thought. The estimated number of college students with AD/HD is around 6 to 7 percent. While this is a new area of research and little is known, preliminary studies of a small group of college students with AD/HD have found that these students have lower grade point averages and are on academic probation more than non-AD/HD peers. Fewer adults with AD/HD complete college: 18 percent compared to 26 percent of adults without AD/HD.

What does the employment future look like for AD/HD children?

When children continue to have AD/HD in their adult years, the struggles they had in school show up on the job. Troubles focusing, organizing work, completing tasks, and making repeated careless mistakes are typical of the AD/HD adult employee. So too are problems getting along with co-workers, accepting direction and feedback from supervisors, and even getting to work on time.

The result is that the adult with AD/HD changes jobs more frequently than non-AD/HD adults. On the average, they have 5.4 jobs in a ten-year period compared to their nondisordered counterparts who have an average of 3.4. More than 40 percent of adults with AD/HD say their symptoms have played a role in their losing, or voluntarily leaving, a job. Frequent job changes mean periodic unemployment. On the average, 52 percent of adults with AD/HD are employed at any given time, compared with 72 percent of non-AD/HD adults.

Difficulty in the workforce can translate into lower income. On the average, adults with AD/HD who graduate high school have average household incomes $10,000 per year lower than non-AD/HD high school graduates. Of those AD/HD adults who graduate college, their income is at least $4,000 per year lower than non-AD/HD college graduates.

What types of careers are AD/HD children likely to succeed in?

The severity of symptoms and coexisting disorders will have a significant impact on the career choice and success a child with AD/HD ultimately has. The range of successful careers found in the AD/HD population is as wide ranging as the non-AD/HD population.

Many go on to become physicians, lawyers, and psychologists. Artists, musicians, actors, and comedians have their share of AD/HD adults.

For the student who is not college bound, technical and trade schools offer good career opportunities. These schools are short-term, hands-on, involve physical activity, and have limited book work, making it the ideal learning environment for those who still have symptoms.

Research has found that many adults who retain symptoms of AD/HD eventually own their own small business. Their difficulties getting along with others, following rules and instructions, meeting deadlines, and managing their time has been found to be less problematic when they work for and by themselves. The variety of independent businesses are vast, yet there is a trend of AD/HD adults pursuing careers in house painting, home repair and maintenance, plumbing, construction, auto mechanics, landscaping, pool cleaning, and similar trades that tend to be more accepting of less predictability in work performance.

What is the risk for AD/HD children to smoke?

Studies have consistently found that children with AD/HD are more at risk for smoking in their teen years than children without these disorders. Those with the most severe attention problems appear to be at the highest risk. When Conduct Disorder coexists with AD/HD, the rate of cigarette smoking increases to as much as five times the rate of teens with AD/HD alone.

Almost twice as many teens with AD/HD smoke cigarettes compared to their nondisordered peers. Most try their first cigarette an average of two years earlier than their non-AD/HD peers. Those teens who continued to have AD/HD were twice as likely to smoke as those who no longer had the disorder.

Teens with AD/HD have an earlier progression to daily smoking and are twice as likely to become daily smokers as their non-AD/HD smoking peers. These findings continue into adulthood. As teens who smoke mature into adulthood, studies find that close to 40 percent of males and females who still have AD/HD continue to smoke. Once they become regular smokers, adults with AD/HD have a more difficult time quitting. Adult males who continue to have AD/HD quit smoking at a considerably lower rate than their non-AD/HD male counterparts.

What is the risk for AD/HD children to use alcohol?

Alcohol is the most frequently used substance in the USA. Anywhere from 66 to 90 percent of adults report having consumed alcohol at least once. Over 8 percent of all adults are dependent on alcohol. In stark comparison, about one third of adults with AD/HD are thought to abuse alcohol.

Alcohol is the most commonly used substance among teens. Children diagnosed with AD/HD have been found to be more at risk for using alcohol in their teen years than their nondiagnosed peers.

Studies have found that children with the most severe problems with attention were at the highest risk. Surprisingly, problems with paying attention appear to be a better predictor than behavior problems. Researchers hypothesize that this may be due to the effect that attention problems have on academic performance and social relationships, which may work together to lead the teen to a nonconformist peer group who accepts the use and abuse of alcohol.

Teens that still have AD/HD in their adolescent years report more drunkenness from alcohol and more alcohol problems than teens without a childhood history of AD/HD.

Those teens with AD/HD who go on to develop severe conduct problems are found to have the highest levels of drinking alcohol.

What is the risk for AD/HD children to use drugs?

It is common knowledge that individuals with significant psychological problems have a higher risk for substance use, abuse, and dependence. AD/HD clearly holds its own risk. Of adolescents referred for substance abuse disorder treatment, roughly one third have AD/HD.

Not surprisingly, the risk for using drugs in adolescence is higher for teens with AD/HD. Not only are they more likely to use drugs, they use them at an earlier age than their nondisordered peers. This represents a serious concern, as the age of first substance use is a well-established predictor of later problematic use.

Variety of drug use is also increased among teens with AD/HD. Twenty percent of teens with AD/HD report using at least one other drug besides marijuana, compared to only 7 percent of teens without AD/HD.

Teens with AD/HD who use drugs have a much higher rate of developing a substance abuse disorder. The general population has a rate of 3 to 5 percent of teenagers with substance abuse disorders.

In contrast, teens with AD/HD have a much higher rate, with some studies estimating more than 35 percent for boys and greater than 15 percent for girls.

School failure, depression, and antisocial peer groups significantly increase the risk for AD/HD children to use and abuse drugs.

What factors increase the risk of drug use in teens with AD/HD?

Initial studies on the relationship between AD/HD and substance abuse found a strong correlation. For years, AD/HD was viewed as a serious risk factor for substance abuse in adolescence. However, as research progresses, the picture of how these two disorders relate has become more clear.

Recent findings have pointed to the addition of Conduct Disorder as a key factor that increases substance abuse in AD/HD teens. One study found that adolescents with both AD/HD and CD had a rate of substance abuse of 59 percent while those with AD/HD alone had a rate of only 4 percent. Teens with both AD/HD and CD have higher rates of substance use and abuse than AD/HD alone or CD alone. Males and females who engage in stealing, defying parents, lying, and starting fights with peers are known to have higher rates of alcohol problems and to have the most severe substance abuse disorders.

Simply having AD/HD alone does not appear to be as strongly correlated with substance use or abuse as previously thought. Other risk factors associated with AD/HD such as academic failure, family stress, poor self-esteem, and poor peer relationships are also thought to cause a predisposition toward drug and alcohol use.

What is the risk for drug use in adults with AD/HD?

The actual risk of trying an illicit drug at least once has been found by some studies to be equal—with 52 percent of adults with AD/HD and 52 percent of non-AD/HD adults reporting having used drugs recreationally.

However, drug abuse in adults with AD/HD is higher than in the general population. Two percent of adults in the U.S. have a drug abuse disorder. Yet, 10 to 20 percent of the adult population with AD/HD has an addictive disorder. Many of these adults report that their addiction began in adolescence or during their young-adult years. The average age of onset of a substance abuse disorder for those with AD/HD is nineteen years.

As with adolescent substance abuse treatment programs, a high number of adults in drug rehabilitation programs have AD/HD. Forty percent of cocaine and opiate abusers are reported to have a history of AD/HD. Compared to other opiate and cocaine abusers, those with a history of AD/HD tended to begin their drug abuse at an earlier age, had more severe abuse habits, and had higher rates of criminal and antisocial behavior.

Are there factors that reduce the risk of drug use?

The good news is that most children with AD/HD do not develop substance abuse disorders. While the statistics cited above are indeed alarming, they still shed light on the fact that more children with AD/HD remain free of substance abuse than those who develop disorders.

Factors that may reduce the risk for drug use and abuse are not well-known. One reason for this lack of understanding is that the idea of treating children with AD/HD throughout their childhood and adolescence is relatively new. Thus, there is only scant research on what long-term treatment can actually do.

One of the more promising findings comes from a group of six studies that followed AD/HD children into adolescence and found that those who were not treated with medication were over three times more likely to develop a substance abuse disorder. These findings suggest that treatment with medication may decrease the risk for substance abuse disorders. The reasons for these findings are not clear; however, researchers are hypothesizing that the medicated children may have found greater success in school, behavior, and social relationships, and were therefore less likely to turn to drugs.

What is the risk of acting out behavior for AD/HD teens?

Acting out behavior refers to aggressive, defiant, irresponsible, and minor illegal activities. For some teens, acting out behavior is a preview of more serious antisocial and criminal behavior to later surface. Impulsivity results in problematic behavior that can surface in any arena of the teenager's life. Troubles with family, friends, and sexual partners are seen more often in AD/HD teens than their nondisordered counterparts.

Twice as many teens with AD/HD will run away from home than teens without AD/HD. About 16 percent of all teens run away from home at some point compared to 32 percent of teens with AD/HD.

AD/HD teens are sexually impulsive. They are ten times more likely to either get pregnant or cause a pregnancy than those without AD/HD. Teens with AD/HD are four times more likely to contract a sexually transmitted disease than teens without AD/HD. Sixteen percent of AD/HD teens contract a sexually transmitted disease while only 4 percent of non-AD/HD teens do.

Predictors of acting out and juvenile delinquency from highest to lowest include drug use, stealing, childhood aggression, childhood behavior problems, truancy, suspension or expulsion from school, maladjustment in elementary school, low educational achievement, and lying.

What is the sexual behavior of AD/HD teens and adults?

Parents tend to be in denial and are surprised to find that almost 47 percent of all high school students have had sexual intercourse at least once. One in five teens in the U.S. has had sexual intercourse before his or her 15th birthday. The earlier teens start having sex, the more partners they have, the more sexually transmitted diseases they contract, and the more pregnancies they cause or experience. For girls who begin sexual activity before the age of fourteen, there is the added risk of dropping out of high school.

While sexual activity does not cause acting out behaviors, teens that have engaged in sex are more likely to smoke cigarettes, drink alcohol, and use drugs. More than 40 percent of teens who had sex at least once had also smoked marijuana, compared with only 10 percent of sexually inexperienced teens.

For AD/HD teenagers, sexual behavior presents the same types of risk, just at a much higher frequency. AD/HD teens generally have more partners, more unprotected sex, more sexually transmitted diseases, and are more likely to become pregnant or cause a pregnancy. The same pattern follows in adulthood. Impulsivity, failure to think of consequences, and need for novelty are likely contributors.

What are the chances for AD/HD teens and adults to engage in crime?

Teens with AD/HD are significantly more likely to have adversarial contacts with law enforcement agencies, 19 percent of AD/HD adolescents compared to 3 percent of non-AD/HD teens. These AD/HD teens are also more likely to be admitted to juvenile justice facilities at a rate of five times more often than non-AD/HD peers. Estimates range from 20 percent to as high as 50 percent of teens in juvenile justice facilities having AD/HD.

Teens that have never had any form of treatment for their AD/HD have been found to average two arrests by the age of eighteen. Those who have had treatment have far less risk for arrest.

Adults with AD/HD are twice as likely to have been arrested as non-AD/HD adults. Estimates are that 37 percent of adults with AD/HD have at least one arrest. Over the past three decades, the chances of ever going to prison has tripled for males and increased sixfold for females. Almost 2 percent of American adult females and 11 percent of adult males will serve time in prison. Presently about one in every thirty-seven adults in the U.S. has served time in prison. While we tend to think of criminal activity as a young man's behavior, the truth is that males ages thirty-five to thirty-nine have the highest risk of going to prison. Those with AD/HD have even greater odds of finding themselves incarcerated. As many as 50 percent of men in prison have a history of AD/HD.

While AD/HD is a factor in crime, in and of itself it has little connection. Criminal behavior in adolescence and adulthood most often occurs in the context of drug abuse.

When determining which AD/HD children will turn to drugs and criminal behavior, it seems that a history of childhood and adolescent aggressive behavior is the main distinguishing factor. The more severe the aggressive behavior is, the stronger the connection to substance abuse and criminal behavior. The age of onset also contributes to later criminal behavior, with those who are severely aggressive at a young age having the higher risk.

What is the risk for auto accidents for AD/HD teens and adults?

Driving is a rite of passage that teens come to expect as their birthright. Serious accidents and fatalities caused by teen drivers have led many states to tighten the restrictions on licensed teenagers. Males between age sixteen and twenty-five are the most dangerous drivers on the road. They become even more dangerous when AD/HD is added. Inattention, distractibility, poor concentration, and impulsivity increase the risk of accidents for AD/HD drivers.

Studies indicate that teens with AD/HD are three times more likely to have driven a vehicle before receiving their driver's permit. They do this nine times more often than their non-AD/HD peers. Teens with AD/HD have their driver's license suspended or revoked at a significantly higher rate than non-AD/HD adolescents.

Teens with AD/HD receive four times the traffic tickets of their non-AD/HD peers, mostly for speeding. They cause and experience four times more automobile accidents and sustain more bodily injuries in those accidents than other drivers.

Driving habits do not improve after high school. One study found college students with a high level of AD/HD symptoms experienced more aggressive and risky driving behavior. They also displayed more driving anger and displayed that anger in hostile, aggressive, and socially inappropriate ways.

What is the likelihood of AD/HD teens developing Antisocial Personality Disorder?

Antisocial Personality Disorder (ASPD) is diagnosed only after age eighteen years and after a pattern of antisocial behavior has been established in adolescence. Individuals with ADHD are about seven times more likely to develop ASPD. However, the ADHD alone has little correlation. The addition of Conduct Disorder to ADHD increases the risk dramatically. Those with ADD are not at risk for developing ASPD as they lack the impulsivity and hyperactivity so often associated with ASPD.

The path from ADHD to ASPD appears to be a predictable one that begins with an early onset of Oppositional Defiant Disorder coexisting with ADHD. Early childhood is plagued by defiance, oppositional behavior, and tantrums. Mid to late childhood is marked by aggression, lying, stealing, and conflicts with the family. When the ODD and ADHD persist into adolescence, Conduct Disorder blossoms into increasingly antisocial behaviors, which ultimately culminates in ASPD in adulthood.

Family factors, environment, genetics, and substance abuse determine the chances that this path will be followed. The greatest predictor of antisocial behavior in adulthood is found in those children who have the earliest onset of antisocial behavior in childhood. In the general population, about 3 percent of males and 1 percent of females have ASPD. In the ADHD population, estimates as high as 25 percent have been reported.

What are the chances of my child having a successful marriage?

The limited findings reveal that adults with AD/HD report general marital unhappiness, less family satisfaction, lower emotional involvement, and less communication. Their non-AD/HD spouses report a plethora of problems caused by the AD/HD spouse, leading to a divorce rate of twice the general population.

Spouses report that their AD/HD partner interferes with household organization, time management, child rearing, and communication. The AD/HD spouses are reported to poorly manage finances, have a poor sense of time, procrastinate on household duties, and rarely initiate helping around the house. Spouses report having to take over household duties, manage appointments, and give frequent reminders of what needs to be done.

Problems with intimacy and expressing feelings are reported by spouses due to frequent arguments, misunderstandings, and lack of support. Their AD/HD partners often fail to follow through on promises and commitments.

An alarming 40 percent of spouses report that their AD/HD partner has trouble getting along with coworkers, is poorly organized at work, and appears lazy to coworkers and supervisors.

AD/HD adults who are in school while married are reported by their spouses to need significant help with studies. Spouses take on the role of explaining concepts, organizing homework, and making sure assignments are turned in.

What kind of parents do AD/HD adults make?

On the heels of not being the ideal spouse, adults who continue to have AD/HD are often weak in their parenting abilities. Because the majority of individuals with AD/HD are male, the father is usually the less effective parent.

Non-AD/HD spouses found their AD/HD partners to quickly lose their temper with their children, be inconsistent with discipline, and to become easily frustrated. Nondisordered parents often have to protect their child from the AD/HD parent's blowups.

Poor judgment in parenting has also been reported in terms of impulsive decisions related to the children. Adults with AD/HD are reported to engage in excessively rough play with their child and the non-AD/HD spouse has to calm the child down after the AD/HD parent wound him up.

AD/HD adults are reported to frequently forget important child-rearing activities and prefer to be an entertaining parent rather than sharing the discipline with their spouse.

Non-AD/HD spouses tend to take over all childrearing activities, including appointments, discipline, homework, carpooling, and communicating with teachers.

Interestingly, even though the spouses reported having to do the majority of the childrearing, their reported levels of marital satisfaction are higher than their AD/HD spouse.

What is the risk for AD/HD children to develop emotional problems as an adult?

Children who outgrow AD/HD by the end of adolescence have an equal chance as anyone to have a happy adulthood. Individuals who continue to have the disorder into their adult years are at risk for emotional difficulties.

Adults with AD/HD are three times more likely than their nondisordered counterparts to experience significant stress, depression, or other emotional problems. Their overall level of functioning tends to be impaired. The more symptoms they have, the more difficulty they have. Twenty-four percent of adults with AD/HD report missing an average of eleven days per month of important activities, such as work, due to their symptoms and related problems. Only 9 percent of the non-AD/HD adults report this same alarmingly high rate of failure to function.

College students with AD/HD exhibit significantly higher levels of anger in their personality. They experience more episodes of anger and show more dysfunctional and socially inappropriate ways of expressing it. Overall, these young adults have more symptoms of psychological distress, more difficulty in interpersonal relations, and more labile, anxious, and depressed moods than non-AD/HD peers.

What can parents do to ensure a good future for their child?

Every parent wants his or her child to be happy and have a successful life. As a parent of an AD/HD child, you have a far greater challenge than other parents. You are the key to your child's happiness and success. The more help you provide your child, the greater his chance for a happy childhood and adolescence, and for a good future as an adult. You have a responsibility to do all you can for your child. Having a child with AD/HD means sacrificing time, effort, emotions, and money to give your child the best life possible.

As a parent of an AD/HD child, the first step to take to help your child is to acknowledge the difficulty you are faced with and accept that you need professional guidance. You are not expected to know how to raise a child with a disorder. There is no shame in getting help, only in refusing to admit that you need it.

What AD/HD children need:

- A thorough evaluation
- Other disorders diagnosed or ruled out
- Section 504 accommodations and modifications
- Behavior modification
- Social skills training
- Anger management training
- Emotion regulation training
- Decision making training
- Extracurricular activities

What AD/HD children might need:

- Tutoring
- Special education
- Individual psychotherapy
- Medication
- Family therapy

Can AD/HD be a strength?

Despite the large number of problems that necessitates psychotherapy, AD/HD does not have to be completely negative. Some children with AD/HD are able to embrace their symptoms and find the unique benefits the disorder offers. When parents and children change their perspective, some of the symptoms of AD/HD can become assets to be harnessed instead of symptoms to try to eliminate.

AD/HD children often have a very unique way of perceiving things. They think of things that no one else could ever possibly entertain. Today's business model of "thinking outside the box" is made for the AD/HD person. While schools may not value the entrepreneurial spirit of an AD/HD child, there are many arenas outside of school that do.

List the symptoms your child exhibits and consider how each might be channeled into a talent, hobby, or strength. Video game obsession can be developed into a hobby through graphic arts and computer classes. A bizarre sense of humor can find a home in comedy and acting workshops. Socially isolated children who find solace in books can make social connections in a book club.

Turning a symptom into a strength can change the way you respond to your child. Your child will find increased happiness and esteem from this approach.

What is the good news about AD/HD?

The future of your child may look rather bleak at first glance of the research findings. School failure, poor social relationships, smoking, drugs, alcohol, and car accidents, among the other negative outcomes, paint a rather grim outlook. Meant to inform rather than depress you as a parent, these statistics provide you with the harsh reality of what can happen to your child. These findings should prompt you into action to obtain all the services your child needs and to stick with them for as long as your child is displaying symptoms.

While the statistics bring bad news, they simultaneously bring good news.

Approximately:

- 30 percent of children with AD/HD no longer have the disorder as a teen.
- 68 percent do not run away from home.
- 87 percent graduate high school.
- 87 percent do not engage in multi-drug use.
- 66 percent do not abuse alcohol.
- 65 percent of boys and 86 percent of girls do not develop a drug abuse disorder.
- 60 percent who smoke cigarettes quit by adulthood.
- 80 percent of teens do not engage in criminal behavior.
- 63 percent of adults with AD/HD do not engage in criminal activities.

The good news is that with treatment and your diligent efforts your child has a good chance of having a positive outcome.

Can AD/HD be a gift?

It's all in how you look at it. The more you and your child can view the symptoms in a positive way, the less negative impact the disorder will have. Your child's qualities and his day-to-day life actually sound rather pleasant if you view your child's symptoms as a gift.

Symptom	Gift
• Impulsive	• Lives fully in the moment
• Hyperactive	• Energetic
• Daydreaming	• Gets into state of relaxation
• Distractible	• Attends to the unobserved in the world
• Forgetful	• Free from endless list of things to do
• Loses things	• Unbound by material things
• Acts like does not hear	• Easily tunes out annoying stimuli/people
• Talks too much	• Passionate about ideas/interests
• Interrupts	• Excited to share ideas with others
• Repeats same mistake	• Not plagued with guilt for mistakes
• Hates homework	• Incredible capacity for play
• Distorted reality testing	• Unique view of the world
• Obsessed	• Passionate
• Ignores others	• Single-mindedness of purpose
• Bizarre sense of humor	• Unique sense of humor
• Selfish	• Gets own needs met
• Greedy	• Strong desires for more
• Pushy	• Doing what it takes to get more
• No self-awareness	• Free from self-consciousness
• Lack of insight	• Free from preoccupation with own faults
• Focuses on irrelevant	• Finds entertainment in mundane things

Appendix A

THE 5 MOST IMPORTANT LISTS YOU NEED

10 Questions You Must Ask Your Doctor about Diagnosis

1. Is AD/HD an area of specialty for you?
2. What procedures do you use to evaluate for AD/HD?
3. Do you think all children need to have formal testing to be evaluated?
4. Will you use psychological testing? If so, what tests and what is the purpose?
5. Do you use medical tests? If so, what tests and what is the purpose?
6. What sources of information do you use to make your diagnosis?
7. How do you distinguish ordinary behavior from AD/HD?
8. What other disorders will you consider besides AD/HD?
9. Will you review my child's school records?
10. Are there indications that my child should be tested for learning disorders?

10 Coexisting Disorders Your Doctor Must Consider

1. Learning Disorders
2. Oppositional Defiant Disorder
3. Conduct Disorder
4. Depression
5. Anxiety
6. Tourette's Disorder
7. Asperger's Disorder
8. Obsessive Compulsive Disorder
9. Bipolar Disorder
10. Encopresis and Enuresis

10 Things You Must Tell Your Child's Teacher

1. That your child has AD/HD
2. Whether or not your child has other diagnoses
3. Whether or not your child has any learning disorders
4. If your child is from a divorced family
5. If your child has toileting issues
6. What behavior problems can be expected in the classroom
7. What behavior problems can be expected on the playground
8. What rewards your child is motivated to work for
9. What consequences are effective in decreasing inappropriate behavior
10. What special talents, hobbies, and interests your child has

10 Parenting Techniques You Must Use

1. Structured routine
2. Rules and rule notebook
3. Consequences
4. Consistency
5. Praise
6. Rewards
7. Behavior chart
8. Predictable consequences
9. Time-out
10. Contracts

10 Questions You Must Ask Your Doctor about Medication

1. How familiar are you with this medication?
2. What is the main purpose of this medication?
3. Is this medication approved for my child's age?
4. What are the side effects of this medication?
5. How often will you see my child to monitor his response to the medication?
6. Are you available for emergency contact if my child has a serious reaction?
7. Do you have written information to give me about this medication?
8. What are the pros and cons of taking this medication only on school days?
9. How should I monitor for side effects?
10. Do you believe in giving multiple medications?

SECTION 504 ACCOMMODATION AND MODIFICATIONS

Section 504 Accommodations and Modifications

This chart may be used in several ways. You may use it to prepare for your Section 504 meeting by identifying which symptoms your child has that interfere with his ability to benefit from his education. Review the list of possible accommodations and modifications and choose those that you feel may be of help to your child. Bring this sheet with you to your meeting as a worksheet when working with your child's education team.

If you are not seeking Section 504 accommodations and modifications, but would like to work with your child's teacher to implement a few of the ideas listed here, you may bring this worksheet with you to your parent-teacher conference as a tool you both can use to find solutions.

Whether or not your child has Section 504, you can use this worksheet for yourself. Follow the same steps of identifying the symptoms and implementing some of the suggested accommodations and modifications at home. These techniques work anywhere, not just in the classroom.

Finally, you may use this chart in your work with your child's psychologist. Learning how to execute many of these techniques is easier said than done. Professional guidance can help you fine-tune your skills and allow you to rapidly find success.

Try to select a realistic number of techniques. Try as you might, it would be impossible to do them all! Focus on one to three techniques until you have them solidly in place before adding more. Over time, you will be able to employ many of these techniques to structure how you work with your child and her school work. As she matures, changes from grade to grade, and circumstances change, you will need to modify the techniques you use to fit her level of functioning and her unique home and school situation.

SYMPTOM	ACCOMMODATION/ MODIFICATION
Difficulty sequencing and completing steps to accomplish longer-term projects such as book reports and term papers.	• Break task into small steps. • Provide written step-by-step instructions. • Allow additional time to complete project • Set deadline for each step
Shifting from one uncompleted activity to another.	• Tell exactly what must be done before changing tasks, "you must finish A, then you can start B." • Praise at completion of each task. • Re-direct to finish incomplete tasks. • Remind what reward awaits at completion.
Difficulty following through on instructions. Seems not to listen when spoken to.	• Gain attention before giving directions. • Use alerting cues before giving directions • Pair oral directions with written directions. • Give one direction at a time. . • Quietly repeat directions to the student. • Have child repeat the directions. • Praise when directions are followed. • Use simple instructions. • Use instruction on exactly what to do and how.

Difficulty prioritizing assignments and tasks.	• Prioritize assignments/tasks for the child. • Provide written list of what to do in order. • Assist child in determining priority. • Praise for appropriate prioritizing.
Difficulty sustaining effort.	• Reduce assignment length. • Grade on accuracy not quantity. • Frequent praise for effort. • Make task interesting • Involve physical activity if possible • Use novelty to increase interest • Remind what reward awaits at completion
Difficulty completing assignments.	• Provide written step-by-step instructions. • Break assignment into small steps. • Assign time for completion of each step. • Make frequent checks during assignment.
Difficulty with test taking.	• Allow extra time to take test. • Provide instruction on test-taking skills. • Allow student to be tested orally. • Allow ample space to write responses.
Difficulty taking notes during classroom instruction and lecture.	• Provide child with a copy of teacher's notes. • Allow student to share notes with peer. • Allow use of tape recorder. • Teacher to emphasize key points

Easily distracted by extraneous stimuli.	• Praise for paying attention. • Break up activities into small units. • Reward for timely accomplishments. • Use physical proximity and touch. • Use preferential seating to be near teacher. • Remove distractions. • Sit near quiet peer. • Provide quiet place to work if child chooses.
Poor organization and planning.	• Teach organizational skills • Establish weekly notebook checks • Create bin for returning homework. • Give extra credit for neatness. • Allow use of computer instead of writing. • Allow use of wide-lined paper.
Poor handwriting.	• Grade for content, not handwriting. • Allow use of a computer instead of writing. • Allow for voice recognition software. • Allow printing instead of handwriting.
Careless errors and repeated mistakes.	• Prompt student to check work. • Return assignments for child to correct. • Allow credit for corrected errors. • Cue child to look for his common errors. • Allow extra time to check for errors. • Allow study buddy to check for errors.

Takes excessive time to complete homework.	<ul><li>Allow alternative method to complete homework, e.g. oral presentation, taped report, visual presentation, etc.</li><li>Reduce amount of writing required.</li><li>Allow for typing.</li><li>Allow for voice recognition software.</li><li>Reduce amount of assignment.</li><li>Set finite time to work on homework.</li><li>Grade for mastery of information, not quantity.</li><li>Give homework for entire week ahead of time.</li></ul>
Inattentive, daydreaming.	<ul><li>Gain attention before giving directions.</li><li>Prompt child to pay attention.</li><li>Prompt child to make eye contact.</li><li>Ask child to repeat directions or information.</li><li>Actively involve student in lesson.</li><li>Make task/assignment interesting.</li><li>Remind what reward awaits.</li><li>Use physical touch to gain attention.</li><li>Get physically close to gain attention.</li><li>Physically lower yourself to child's eye level.</li></ul>
Talkative, disruptive to class, and difficulty working quietly.	<ul><li>Seat child near teacher.</li><li>Catch child being good and praise</li><li>Use hand signal to prompt child to remain quiet.</li><li>Use behavior chart for remaining in seat.</li><li>Use behavior chart for working quietly.</li><li>Quietly praise child for being quiet.</li></ul>

Inappropriate seeking of attention.	• Ignore minor misbehavior. • Teach how to obtain attention appropriately. • Praise quickly when child is appropriate. • Use time-out when inappropriate. • Give re-direction of how to behave.
Difficulty making transitions between activities.	• Warn prior to transition. • Post routine of activities on wall. • Assign buddy to accompany child during transitions. • Remind child how to behave during transition.
Difficulty remaining seated and excessively physically active.	• Give frequent opportunities to get out of seat. • Allow space at desk for movement. • Allow standing at desk.
Frequent fidgeting with hands, feet, or objects; squirming in seat.	• Allow movement when possible. • Ignore minor movements. • Prompt for child to sit still. • Praise child for sitting still. • Provide an object to fidget with.
Blurts out answers in class.	• Seat child near teacher. • Prompt child to raise hand. • Prompt child to wait question is finished. • Praise child for raising hand. • Inform student when you will call on him, e.g. "I will call on Mary, then James, and then Cameron you will have your turn." • Praise student for being patient.

Difficulty waiting turn, intrusive, and interrupts others.	• Prompt student to wait turn. • Praise student when he waits his turn. • Provide empathy about waiting being difficult.
Insistent on getting own way.	• Provide empathy about not getting own way. • Teach appropriate way to get needs met. • Teach child how to compromise. • Set firm limit when child cannot have his way. • Warn of consequence if insistence continues. • Praise when child he accepts not getting his way.
Difficulty using unstructured time on playground, hallways, lunchtime, library time, etc.	• Post rules on classroom wall. • Prompt for exactly what behavior is expected. • Help child select activity ahead of time. • Assign buddy to accompany child. • Define consequences of rule breaking. • Praise appropriate behavior. • Create a reward system for appropriate behavior.
Forgetful.	• Post daily routine on wall • Post rules on wall • Create checklist of "To Do"

Losing things necessary for task or activities at school or at home.	• Help child keep tack of belongings each day. • Daily checking of notebook/backpack for young children. Weekly for older children. • Praise child for keeping track of items. • Provide checklist of items and their location. • Set up child's notebook, backpack, closet, etc. • Color code books, notebooks, flash cards. • Use color coded and labeled bins for items. • Use Velcro sealed plastic pouch for homework.
Poor use of time.	• Use secret signal to prompt child to do work. • Set time line to complete a small assignment. • Frequent praise for working. • Praise completion of work. • Use a timer to "race" against. • Provide reward/privilege when work is complete.

BEHAVIOR CHARTS

The Weekly Behavior Chart

The Weekly Behavior Chart is to be used for children with only minor behavior problems or those who are incapable of a comprehensive behavior program that addresses multiple behaviors.

Select three behaviors that your child wants to work on to earn rewards. Discuss with your child rewards that he would like to earn each day for completing each of the three tasks. The rewards should be small but motivating enough to get him excited about cooperating. For each behavior he successfully completes, he earns one reward, giving him three possible rewards to earn each day. He must be given the earned rewards each day he earns them. If you fail to give him his daily reward, he will quickly lose motivation, just as you would lose motivation to go to work if your boss did not give you your paycheck.

At the end of the week, if he has completed seven out of seven days, he earns a bigger reward for 100 percent success. Some tasks, such as homework, may only be assigned five days, so he earns his big weekly reward if he is successful five out of five days. Friday or Saturday is a good day to give the weekly rewards.

BEHAVIOR	SAT	SUN	MON	TUES	WED	THUR	FRI	WEEKLY REWARD
Do homework by dinner								
Ice cream for dessert								*Go out for pizza*
Turn off video game when told								
25 cents towards new game								*Rent video game*
Brush teeth without argument								
30 minutes of television								*Donuts for breakfast on Sat*

The Daily Behavior Chart

The Daily Behavior Chart is to be used for children who have frequent difficulty following rules and are oppositional and defiant. You can make your own chart, adding and deleting tasks to fit your child. Post the chart where your child can easily see it. Use clip art for each task if your child cannot read or is more visually oriented.

Encourage your child to check his chart frequently to prompt him to do his next task. For very oppositional children, you can make each task worth four points if he complies without arguing. If he argues, then he only earns one point. Outright refusal or failure to cooperate earns a zero.

Bedtime is a nice time to cuddle and review the chart while praising your child for each task she completed. When discussing the tasks she did not complete or argued about, be sure to talk gently. Go over the tasks not completed and encouragingly ask what she thinks she could do differently tomorrow to earn those points. Remain encouraging that tomorrow is a new day and a chance for her to earn more points. Review her point bank so she knows how many points she has saved.

In order for the Daily Behavior Chart to work, you must do it every day without fail. You must remain a cheerleader for your child to follow the chart. Behavior charts that do not work can usually be traced to parents' failure to give the points each day and failure to give rewards when earned. If you are too tired to fill in the chart, how can you expect your child to have the energy to do all the tasks you are asking.

Create your own Reward List by asking your child what she would like to earn. Be sure to list the television, telephone, Internet, video games, movies, toys, and food treats. These are powerful motivational tools that your child is excited to earn. If you give them to her without charging points, you are left with little reason for her to cooperate.

Give plenty of chances for your child to earn points. You want her to realize that if she cooperates, she will be amply rewarded. She should earn enough points so she can spend some each day for daily privileges and treats. She should also be able to earn enough points to save them for bigger privileges and rewards. Use the Bank Sheet each time she earns and spends points.

TASK	TIME	SAT	SUN	MON	TUE	WED	THUR	FRI	WEEK TOTAL
Wake up	6:30AM								
Out of bed	6:45AM								
Get dressed	7:00AM								
Eat breakfast	7:15AM								
Brush teeth	7:30AM								
In car w/ backpack	7:45AM								
Good school day	3:00PM								
Homework	4:00PM								
Good day care	5:00PM								
Pick up @ day care	5:30PM								
Set table	6:00PM								
Eat dinner	6:30PM								
Clear table	7:00PM								
Bath	7:15PM								
Free time	7:45PM								
Bed time	8:15PM								
Lights out	8:30PM								
No time outs									
Share toys									
Turn off computer									
Feed dog AM									
Water dog AM									
Use nice words									
Bonus									
Bonus									
Bonus									
Bonus									
Bonus									
DAILY TOTAL									
1 pt. per behavior									
4 pts. if no arguing									

EDUCATIONAL TESTS

NAME	ACRONYM	PURPOSE	AGE
Wechsler Pre-school and Primary Scale of Intelligence III	WPPSI III	Intelligence (IQ)	2–6 years
Wechsler Intelligence Scale for Children	WISC IV	Intelligence (IQ)	6–16 years
Wechsler Adult Intelligence Scale	WAIS III	Intelligence (IQ)	16–89 years
Woodcock Johnson II	Woodcock Johnson II	Academic achievement	2–90+ years
Kaufman Assessment Battery for Children—II	KABC-II	Cognitive ability	3–18 years
Peabody Individual Achievement Test-Revised	PIAT-R	Academic achievement	5–22 years

Appendix E RECOMMENDED READING

Chapter 1: The ABCs of AD/HD

Websites with helpful information for those beginning their journey with AD/HD:

www.adhdinfo.com
www.addresources.org
www.help4adhd.org
www.chadd.org
www.nimh.nih.gov
www.helpforadd.com
www.ashleypsychology.com

Chapter 2: Getting Your Child Evaluated

American Psychiatric Association. *Diagnostic and Statistical Manual of Mental Disorders IV-TR.* Washington, D.C.. American Psychiatric Association. 2000

Manual of mental disorders with diagnostic criteria and descriptions. Written for trained mental health professionals.

Chapter 3: Coexisting Disorders

American Psychiatric Association. *Diagnostic and Statistical Manual of Mental Disorders IV-TR.* Washington, D.C.: American Psychiatric Association. 2000

Manual of mental disorders with diagnostic criteria and descriptions. Written for trained mental health professionals.

Comings, D. *Tourette's Syndrome and Human Behavior.* Duarte, California: Hope Press. 1990
Authoritative textbook on Tourette's. Includes information about AD/HD coexisting with Tourette's.
Learning Disability OnLine: www.ldonline.com
Information on learning disabilities in general, as well as when it coexists with AD/HD.

Chapter 4: Succeeding in School

U.S. Department of Education: www.ed.gov/about/offices/list/osers/
Information on the Office of Special Education and Rehabilitation Services Council for Exceptional Children: www.cec.sped.org
Information about special education including IDEA.
No Child Left Behind U.S. Department of Education: www.ed.gov/nclb/
Information about No Child Left Behind act.
Section 504 U.S. Department of Education Office for Civil Rights: www.ed.gov/about/offices/list/ocr/504faq.html
Information about Section 504.
FAQ about Special Education: www.wrightslaw.com
Comprehensive website written specifically for parents addressing all areas of special education.
Educational Resources Information Center: www.eric.ed.gov
Information about special education.
Reif. S. *How to Reach and Teach Children with ADD/ADHD: Practical Techniques, Strategies, and Interventions.* San Francisco, CA: Jossey-Bass, 2005
Numerous tips for parents and teachers to use with AD/HD children.

Frank, K. and Smith-Rex, S. *ADHD: 102 Practical Strategies for "Reducing the Deficit."* Chapin, South Carolina: Youthlight, Inc. 2001
Numerous tips for parents and teachers to use with AD/HD children.

Chapter 5: Homework

U.S. Department of Education: www.ed.gov/pubs/HelpingStudents
Information about homework, including USDE guidelines for how much homework is recommended.
National Association of Elementary School Principals: www.naesp.org
Information for school principals, including how to develop guidelines for homework.
Brown Center Report on American Education: www.brookings.edu
Statistics on education in the U.S.
Dendy, C. *Teaching Teens with ADD and ADHD: A Quick Reference Guide for Teachers and Parents.* Bethesda, Maryland: Woodbine House. 2000
Excellent guide for both parents and teachers to help teens with school and homework.

Chapter 6: Parenting: Rules, Routines, and Rewards

Trower, T. *The Self-Control Patrol Workbook: Exercises for Anger Management.* Plainview, New York: Childswork/Childsplay. 1995
Fun and quick one-page exercises for children and pre-teens to help increase awareness of anger and how to gain control over it. Can be used by parents, teachers, youth group and scout leaders, or even read by teens alone.

Kaplan, J. Kid Mod: Empowering *Children and Youth through Instruction in the Use of Reinforcement Principles*. Austin, Texas: Pro-Ed. 1996

Fun exercises for children and pre-teens to help them increase awareness of their choices, behavior, and consequences. Can be used by parents, teachers, and youth group and scout leaders.

Vernon, A. *Thinking, Feeling, Behaving: An Emotional Education Curriculum for Adolescents*. Champaign, Illinois: Research Press. 1989

Exercises and topics for discussion with pre-teen and teens. Can be used by parents, teachers, youth group and scout leaders, or even read by teens alone.

Garber, S., Garber, M., and Spizman, R. *Good Behavior: Over 1200 Sensible Solutions to Your Child's Problems from Birth to Age Twelve*. New York: Villard Books. 1987

Easy-to-use reference book of solutions for the most common behavior problems.

Flick, G. *ADD/ADHD Behavior-Change Resource Kit: Ready-to-Use Strategies & Activities for Helping Children with Attention Deficit Disorder*. Somerset, New Jersey: Jossey-Bass. 2002.

Includes numerous ideas for parents and teachers.

Dinkmeyer, D., McKay, G., and Dinkmeyer, D. *The Parent's Handbook: Systematic Training for Effective Parenting (STEP)*. Circle Pines, Minnesota: American Guidance Service. 1997

One of my favorite books on the basic techniques every parent should use.

Glasser, H. and Easley, J. *Transforming the Difficult Child: The Nurtured Heart Approach*. Tucson, Arizona: Howard Glasser. 2002

Warm and nurturing parenting techniques for parents of very difficult children.

Eimers, R. and Aitchison, R. *Effective Parents/Responsible Children: A Guide to Confident Parenting.* New York: McGraw-Hill Book Company. 1977
Another of my favorite books on parenting. Teaches parents how to use the behavior modification techniques psychologists use.

Levy, R., O'Hanlon, B., and Goode, T. *Try and Make Me!: Simple Strategies that Turn off the Tantrums and Create Cooperation.* Rodale. 2001
This is the book to read when nothing else has worked. For parents of the most difficult oppositional and defiant children.

Greenspan, S. and Greenspan, N. *The Essential Partnership: How Parents and Children can Meet the Emotional Challenges of Infancy.* New York, New York: Viking. 1989
An indispensable book for parents to learn psychological techniques to build a strong emotional relationship with their child.

Gordon, T. *Parent Effectiveness Training: The Proven Program for Raising Responsible Children.* New York, New York: Three Rivers Press. 2000
A classic book in parenting and one of the all-time best, in print since 1970. Teaches verbal skills to help parents talk and listen to their child and learn to understand one another, negotiate, and resolve conflicts.

Chidekel, D. *Parents in Charge: Setting Healthy, Loving Boundaries for You and Your Child.* New York, New York: Simon & Schuster: 2002
Insights on how parents' own childhood effects the way they raise their children. Offers excellent suggestions for parents to take charge of disciplining their child.

Chapter 7: Medication

American Academy of Pediatrics website: www.pediatrics.org
Research findings related to AD/HD and medication and other topics related to AD/HD.
CHADD website: www.chadd.org
Fact sheet on medication for AD/HD.
University of Arkansas Medical Sciences website: www.uams.edu
Fact sheet on medication for AD/HD
Ashley Psychology website: www.ashleypsychology.com
Research findings about AD/HD and medication.
National Institute of Mental Health website: www.nimh.nih.gov
Medication information.
Harvard School of Public Health:
   www.hsph.harvard.edu/Organizations/DDIL/stimtics.html
Literature review of the relationship between stimulant medication and tic disorder.
Tourette's Syndrome "Plus": www.tourettesyndrome.net
Information about the relationship between Tourette's, AD/HD, and medication.

Chapter 8: Social Skills

Schab, L. *The You & Me Workbook*. Plainview, New York: Childswork/
   Childsplay. 2001qw
Fun and quick exercises for children and pre-teens to increase social skills. Easy for parents and teachers to use.
Jackson, N., Jackson, D., and Monroe, C. *Getting Along with Others: Teaching Social Effectiveness to Children: Skill Lessons and Activities* Champaign, Illinois: Research Press. 1983.
Lesson plans for teachers or group therapists to use to teach social skills.

Kincher, J. *Psychology for Kids: 40 Fun Tests That Help You Learn about Yourself.* Minneapolis, Minnesota: Free Spirit Publishing, Inc. 1995

Fun exercises for children and teens to increase self-awareness. Parents can give this book to their child to read and use at their leisure.

Zimmerman, T. and Shapiro, L. *Sometimes I Feel Like I Don't Have Any Friends (But Not So Much Anymore): A Self-Esteem Book to Help Children Improve Their Social Skills.* King of Prussia: Pennsylvania: The Center for Applied Psychology, Inc. 1996

Fun short story for parents or teachers to read to children or simply give the book to the child to read on their own.

Berg, B. *The Social Skills Workbook: Exercises to Improve Social Skills.* Dayton, Ohio: Cognitive Therapeutics. 1990

Exercises to be used in a group setting by therapists or teachers to teach social skills.

Berg. B *The Anger Control Workbook: Exercises to Develop Anger Control Skills.* Dayton, Ohio: Cognitive Therapeutics. 1990

Exercises to be used with older children and teens to teach anger recognition and anger management skills. Can be used independently by a motivated teen.

Mannix, D. *Social Skills Activities for Special Children.* West Nyack, New York: Prentice Hall: 1993.

Fun exercises for children to do in class, group therapy, or at home with parents.

American Girl Library. *The Care and Keeping of Friends.* Middleton, Wisconsin: Pleasant Company Publications. 1996.

Fun book for girls to read to improve friendship skills.

American Girl Library. *Oops! The Manners Guide for Girls.* Middleton, Wisconsin: Pleasant Company Publications. 1997.

Fun colorful book for girls to read alone or with their parent.

Delmege, S. *Girl Friends: How to Be Friends Forever.* New York: Scholastic, Inc. 2002.
Fun book to help children and teen girls learn how to be a good friend. Can be read alone or with a parent.

Schab, L. *The Anger Solution Workbook.* Plainview, New York: Childswork/Childsplay. 2001
Fun and quick exercises for children and teens to learn anger management skills. Can be used with teacher, parents, or alone by child.

Carlson, N. *How to Lose All Your Friends.* New York, New York: Viking. 1994.
By far the most requested book by children to have read to them in social skills therapy. A funny book that teaches children why they lose friends.

Freedman, J. *Easing the Teasing. Helping Your Child Cope with Name-Calling, Ridicule, and Verbal Bullying.* Chicago: Contemporary Books. 2002.
Describes a variety of useful techniques for parents to teach their child how to cope with teasing.

Chapter 9: Self-Esteem

Kaufman, G., Raphael, L., and Espeland, P. *Stick up for Yourself: Every Kid's Guide to Personal Power & Positive Self-Esteem.* Free Spirit Publishing: Minneapolis, Minnesota. 1999
Helpful guide for children who are teased to read either alone or with parents.

Sharpiro, L. *Sometimes I Drive My Mom Crazy, but I Know She's Crazy about Me: A Self-Esteem Book for Overactive and Impulsive Children.* Plainview, New York: Childswork/Childsplay. 1995
Fun story every child with AD/HD should read either alone or with their parents.

Shapiro, L. *How to Raise a Child with a High EQ: A Parent's Guide to Emotional Intelligence.* New York, New York: Perennial Currents. 1998
Excellent book for parents that focuses on the emotional life of children.

Chapter 10: Growing Up with AD/HD

International Narcotics Control Board: www.incb.org
Information related to illicit drug use.
National Center for Education Statistics: www.nces.ed.gov
Statistics on completion of high school in the U.S.
Centers for Disease Control and Prevention: www.cdc.gov
Safety and injury information for AD/HD children.
FBI: www.fbi.gov
Statistics on long-term outcome for children and teens with AD/HD.

Index

About the Author

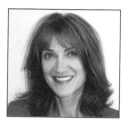 Susan Ashley, PhD is the founder and director of Ashley Children's Psychology Center and has been specializing in ADD and ADHD since 1990. A graduate of UCLA and California School of Professional Psychology, she has over twenty years of education, training, and experience working with children and families. She lives in Northridge, California.